CREATIV

MUSIC

IN GROUPWORK

Dedication

To Dorothy, my wife, who has shared so much with me, and to Murray and Roddy, for putting up with all the writing.

Also to Steve King and Martin Campbell, with gratitude.

'Whatever you can do or dream you can, begin it. Boldness has genius, power and magic in it. Begin it now.' (Goethe)

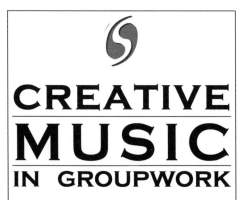

CREATIVE MUSIC IN GROUPWORK

Christopher Achenbach

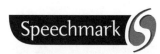

Speechmark Publishing Ltd
Telford Road • Bicester • Oxon OX26 4LQ • UK

Published by
Speechmark Publishing Ltd, Telford Road, Bicester, Oxon OX26 4LQ,
United Kingdom
www.speechmark.net

© C Achenbach, 1997
First published 1997
Reprinted 1998, 2000, 2002

002-2623/Printed in Great Britain/1010

British Library Cataloguing in Publication Data
Achenbach, Chris
    Creative music in groupwork. – (Creative activities in groupwork series)
    1. Music therapy   2. Group psychotherapy
    I. Title
    615.8'5154

ISBN 0 86388 453 9
(Previously published by Winslow Press Ltd under ISBN 0 86388 164 5)

CONTENTS

Chris Achenbach, born in Belfast, is a music therapist and composer who has lived and worked in the Scottish Borders since 1988. He attended Chetham's School, Manchester, then read for a BA in Music at the University of Leeds. He is Music Therapy Manager with Borders Community Health Services (NHS Trust), working in the learning disability and mental health services. His compositions include two short operas with libretti by writer Judy Steel (*Whaup of the Rede* was performed in the 1993 Borders Festival and *Muckle-Mou'd Meg* was premiered in 1995) and other vocal and instrumental works, some of which have been commercially recorded.

His interest in music groupwork stems both from his professional training and experience (he holds a postgraduate diploma from the Nordoff-Robbins Music Therapy Centre, London), and also from joint work with community musicians in a variety of settings over recent years. His teaching commitments include the extra-mural 'Music As Communication' course at the University of St Andrews. Formerly a professional pianist, he loves jazz and has been musical director of the Borders Big Band since 1990. Chris is married to Dorothy, who has three children.

PREFACE

A score is just a score; words are just words. The first is a kind of blueprint for a musical performance, not music in itself. In a similar way, these pages will bear fruit to the extent in which you, the reader, transform them into your own experience. That is where they started for me.

I have no illusions about this manual being definitive. Everyone has good ideas and we should share them when we can. I look forward to hearing those of readers. The field of music groupwork is now home to a whole range of practitioners, many of whom are just starting to discover the value of sharing experience and practice with their peers. They include people from a variety of professional backgrounds, as well as those who do not see themselves as formally skilled or trained (often because such training is not available for them).

I am also happy to notice that my specialization (music therapy) is being welcomed into this wide-ranging company and is not seeking to claim this whole area of work as its own. I am painfully aware that such a charge has been levelled before now. The truth is that both good and bad practice may be found everywhere; what seems more important is to address a common purpose, which (for readers of this book) is to find effective ways of working with others in music. Let us have no snobbery as we try to do this, for we all need to talk to each other. In doing so, and in documenting and evaluating our many ways of working, we will be helping to validate our individual and common methodologies.

I hope you find this book helpful as you make your own creative decisions. Whatever your background and aspirations, I wish you well.

CHRIS ACHENBACH

ACKNOWLEDGEMENTS

The quotation on page 4 is reproduced with kind permission from *Music Therapy: An Art Beyond Words* by Leslie Bunt, published by Routledge.

SECTION 1

THINKING AND PLANNING

Why music?

We are musical because we are human. Like animals, we use sound to communicate our needs and express our emotions. Unlike animals, we have transformed the raw material of sound into something which we call music. What lies behind this transformation?

We do not simply 'live for now' in the way we deduce most animals do. Our minds give us something more: conscious awareness of ourselves as individuals with a past, present and future. Our need to share and test concepts with others has also formed part of our evolution as social beings. Social ritual might, in this context, be considered 'shared conceptualization'. Such ritual appears to help maintain our sense of collective identity. We share grief in bereavement, happiness in producing offspring, suspicion of those who are 'not of us', and hopes and fears about what happens after death.

Music connects with ritual; indeed, its development as an art form is inexorably bound up with it. There is a continuous tradition of music as part of religious worship, from primitive tribal ceremony to Catholic High Mass and Tibetan Buddhist bells, gongs and chants. Spiritual possession and exorcism ceremonies, using fast, repetitive drumming and chanting, are still found, not just in Africa, but also in Brazil, the West Indies and even Protestant churches in the southern United States.

Besides the tribal ceremonies mentioned above, medical ritual and practice has commonly involved music. The ancient Greeks believed the use of certain modes (scales) were beneficial to health, while they proscribed others; Anton Mesmer had the piano played while offering his 'magnetic cures', and modern dentists are rediscovering the analgesic effect of loud music in their surgeries.

Are we really so far from our ancestors' campfires? We surrender our individuality at rock concerts, sing and dance the conga at parties and expect certain 'socially sacred' music at weddings. Musical ritual seems alive and well.

Music is all around us these days. We listen to recorded and (sometimes) live music every day. Our television and radio consumption includes a huge amount of carefully chosen musical material, and the tunes we hear when shopping in a supermarket are thoughtfully selected also. In all this, do we still create music for ourselves? In fact we do, usually without realizing it. The building-blocks of what we define as music are still the sounds and rhythms that we use to express ourselves and communicate with others. A young child learning to speak babbles tunefully to herself, echoing the falling cry of her mother calling her for lunch. Workmen set up a rhythm with picks as they dig. A cattle auctioneer adopts a singsong voice in the hubbub of the market. Soldiers chant while they march. There is still a human use of 'musical' sound which might be seen as 'pre-musical' or unconsciously so.

This directs us towards the effectiveness of music as a therapeutic medium. Leslie Bunt (1994) defines music therapy as 'the organised use of sounds and music within an evolving relationship between client and therapist to support and encourage physical, mental, social and emotional well-being'. Most creative groupwork involves the therapeutic goals familiar to music therapists: expressive freedom, communicative competence, psychological health and the fulfilment of personal potential. Music can also be combined with other art forms (such as drama, movement and art) in these and other models of work.

Therapeutic aims are not the whole story, however; music groupwork can also involve imaginative creation, purposeful collaboration and fun. It can awaken our sense of shared ritual, stimulate us to work creatively with others and help us rediscover ways of expressing ourselves which we sorely need in our arid, inhibited society.

Creative and interactive skills

I suggest two main areas of skill acquisition and development in music groupwork: creative and interactive. Each implies a number of more specific skills which can be developed and enhanced by means of intelligently planned groupwork. Such learning may be seen as experiential: that is to say, taking place within the medium of active/interactive musical experience.

As regards creative skills (Table 1), the first must be our freedom and confidence to choose a sound and explore: to create sound for its own sake. Immersed in such exploration, we can bypass intellectual judgement, leading to the unpremeditated expression of the way we feel at that moment, the nature of such expression depending on whom and where we are. Such a 'jumping-off' process is central to the music improvisation ideas presented in this book.

The elements involved in developing the creative impulse in Table 1 are more than just musical techniques (although they relate to the creation of all types of music, from serious composition to improvised jazz or rock solos). They are also indicators of the intent, creativity and interior psychological territory of the improviser.

With the comparison of depicting and conceptualizing we enter fresh musical and psychological territory. The first suggests a concrete portrayal by means of sound (for example, a thunderstorm), the second a translation through, or of, human experience (the anger of a thunderstorm, or personal anger). There is a major conceptual jump, and hence a learning opportunity, in the relationship between the two.

Table 1   *Some creative skills in music groupwork*

Confidence to explore and express
Choosing a sound Being spontaneous 'Jumping off'
Developing the creative impulse
Establishing (a beat, rhythm, phrase) Elaborating (becoming more complex) Transforming (changing, varying) Contrasting (two different musical components) Juxtaposing Combining Intensifying (increasing energy) Resolving Reflecting Concluding
Depicting/Conceptualizing
Painting with sound Translating experience into sound
Purposefulness
Concentrating Problem-solving
Gaining insight
Awareness of own needs

Purposefulness in Table 1 relates here to the personal discipline of working within a process and/or concentrating on a specific task.

Gaining insight is seen as the ability to increase our self-awareness and sense of 'personal well-being' by engaging in, and reflecting on, a musical experience. This does not necessarily mean the latter has to be 'analysed'; the experience itself can be enough for personal growth. There are, however, many working situations where a skilled helper can facilitate the gaining of insight through participation in groupwork.

Interactive skills (see Table 2) widen the scope of experiential learning to include, not just self, but self in relation to others. Since music is a naturally participative medium, it follows that such skills may usefully be developed in planned groupwork.

Listening and sharing are the key skills here, not just of musical interaction, but of all relationships.

Leading, following and supporting are closely related skills of interaction. The chance to take charge of a group can be an important learning experience, as can the concentration and internal discipline required to take direction from another. To be supported is to require to trust; to support is to ask to be trusted.

The ability to collaborate is an indicator of group cohesion and collective trust.

The lists presented in Tables 1 and 2 may be understood as groups of both skills and experiences. How you use them will depend on the needs of your group members. If specialized groupwork is involved, you should also read Section 4 of this book.

Entries in Section 2 include indications of skills relevant to particular activities.

Planning and running a group

Ideas and models

Be clear from the start what kind of group you are planning. Three models crop up regularly in my work: groups for personal growth, for work with creative and interactive skills, and for the enjoyment and experience of those involved (see 'Format' below).

Your groupwork idea may spring from work you are already involved in or crystallize from a concept (one of mine was to explore the relationship between film/television pictures and music). You may have the freedom to design your group from scratch. I find two processes useful here: first, asking potential members about your idea and, second, checking it with someone whose opinion you trust.

Table 2   *Some interactive skills in music groupwork*

Listening and sharing
Waiting Turn-taking Empathizing Acknowledging Asking Answering Offering Accepting Asserting Interrupting Surprising Challenging Resolving
Leading, following and supporting
Trusting
Collaborating
Planning Achieving Reflecting

Remember that, if you have first-time members, you probably have a clearer idea of the possibilities than they do; you need to communicate these. Be clear that what you *want* to do is something you yourself *can* do (for example, working with issues of personal growth or exploring contemporary pop music). Set yourself and the group up to succeed.

Aims (intent)

Your group's statement of aims or intent (and I think there should always be one) will be linked to your choice of model. Be clear about what you want members to achieve. You may also want to pass on groupwork skills to another person as part of your work. You will find it easier to plan format and process with a 'mission statement' to refer to and work from. It is also a useful tool when evaluating the success of your group during and/or after its run.

It can be beneficial for group members to create a statement of intent, thus 'owning' the responsibility for achieving their aims.

Membership

People usually prefer to choose rather than to be chosen. This is important to bear in mind when working somewhere where staff may be used to 'picking' people for activities. An open session can be a good way of offering your wares. I work regularly in wards and units where, time after time, I find that people who choose to make use of a group then 'own' their decision, making the opportunity more effective for themselves from the very start.

Use your experience and judgment to negotiate the size of the group. I prefer to work with no less than three people, with seven as an optimum size. Some of my groups have to be far larger, often at the expense of individual attention to members' needs. Depending on your circumstances, you may need to refuse membership to some, or to encourage, or even demand it, of others. In such circumstances, have your reasons clear before the event and communicate them positively.

Schedule of meetings

Start and finish! Far too much groupwork is set in motion to run forever with an unchanging membership, especially in institutional settings. It is easy for a new group to become a fixture under these circumstances, killing the chance of a creative outcome. Time-limited groupwork creates its own momentum simply by having a limited lifespan. Even when the group process does not include a final 'product', a limited run of meetings will inform that process by providing a beginning, middle and end to the group's life. Endings may be difficult, but they exist, and without them there can be no new growth.

Whatever your frequency of meeting, try to work out your absences in advance. This makes planning easier, and you may not need to be there every time in any case.

Format

In groupwork with *personal growth* aims, membership will almost certainly be closed at, or near, the start of the group's run. Work usually focuses on exploration of issues of personal and/or shared significance for members (especially on a feelings level). It can be an intense experience for all taking part. Members (and facilitators) need to work together to build a framework of trust (including the assurance of confidentiality) and relationship within which members' needs can be met. Such a framework may be present outside the group as well (for example, in a positively run unit or hospital ward), in which case a facilitated turnover of membership is possible; the group, however, will still exist as an independent and creative entity. It would be exceptional for work like this to be led by anyone but a competent professional.

Work with *creative and interactive skills* can benefit everyone; however, planned groupwork of this kind is likely to concentrate on those who need it most. They can include people with a learning disability and/or a disorder of communication, those with long-term mental health problems and others whom society would commonly view as devalued or deviant, such as substance abusers, prisoners or people in challenging social circumstances. Groups may be closed (and on the whole this is generally preferable) but may also be open to a range of potential members, or even 'drop-in' in style. Work with expressive and interactive skills can (and should) include experiences of personal growth, and it is once again important that the group should be able to trust the competence of the facilitators. Sad to say, the surface appearance and terminology of such work is often borrowed by services who are really only looking for ways to occupy people's time.

Groupwork for the *enjoyment and experience* of those involved covers (like the previous model) a huge range of possibilities. Once again, membership may be on a 'drop-in' or open basis, although members themselves may ask for it to be closed in order to achieve their aims. Success here lies in providing opportunities for creative and purposeful collaboration. This is far removed from simply spending time 'doing music'. Whatever your working circumstances, you can find ways to make membership of such a group not just enjoyable, but meaningful. Although training may not be needed, your intent, experience and expertise are.

See Section 4 for some example formats in special needs work.

Setting

Some groups are tied to a particular building, while others can choose from a variety of meeting-places. Choose a soundproof room, free from distractions. There should be enough room to seat everybody in a circle, with instruments and equipment to hand. Check that furniture will meet the group's needs and that wheelchair access, proximity of toilets and so on are adequate. Good lighting is important, but so is the facility to 'black out' (for vocal work, for example). Check with the janitor and any other staff that you will not be disturbed during proceedings.

Resources

Plan in advance who will supply instruments and equipment. Check these beforehand: that 'decent tape recorder' may turn out to be the kind that used to feed programmes into home computers; instruments may turn out to be toys, or otherwise inadequate for the group's needs. Be cynical about 'it'll be there' promises, or assurances that the video camera will be charged the night before.

The other resources are, of course, human. They include you, any other people in supporting roles and whatever mentor you use to support your work. When working with elderly people or with special needs groups (especially in community settings) you will find that supporters are often volunteers and you may need to develop your vetting skills if approached by such people. Beware of those who want to 'aid the unfortunate'; help them develop a fresh perspective or (failing this) to find the nearest exit. The finest volunteers I have ever worked with are those who were genuinely interested in the business of the group. If working with paid staff, it helps enormously if they, like you, *want* to be there and are not just paid to be present. Talk this over beforehand.

Sort out any transport needs ahead of time. If group members depend on convoluted travel arrangements, be aware of any problems that arise at the start and negotiate accordingly.

Process

This is where your statement of intent bears fruit; you will need it as you put your ideas into practice. The following are some issues to bear in mind:

1 Attention span. The average adult can concentrate fruitfully for around 20 minutes. What is your own span?
2 Staying with activities or moving on. Be sensitive to the dynamic of the group and be ready to amend the 'running order' of your plan.
3 Involving only some members at a time. Do members' skills include those of listening and waiting, or do you need to keep people involved? Can the group work on these skills?

4   Start and finish well. Give the group time to warm up, reflect on what happened in the last meeting and plan for the present group; at the end, to wind down, reflect and (if appropriate) plan for the future. Do not jump straight into, or out of, concentrated work.

5   Giving the group time to grow. People need to get to know each other, establish ground rules, work through any problems of communication and/or participation and learn to trust the group process and each other, before they can function at their creative best. Offer the time and space for this to happen.

6   Work with abilities, not disabilities. This is an important mind-set.

7   Be clear and positive. How do you come across to others – do you 'sabotage yourself' by being diffident, mumbling or otherwise 'putting yourself down'? Watching video evidence can be painful, but educational.

8   Overplanning and 'winging it' are both unnecessary sources of stress. Trying to get through an over-full group agenda is no fun; neither is desperately trying to have a brilliant idea about what to do next. Keep your planning simple and leave lots of room for the creative opportunities which will arise during the group: you cannot use them if your mind is tied up in what you think should happen next.

9   Power and control. Creative participation is *not* a matter of exercising control over others, but of sharing working spaces, skills, insights and achievements. There may be specialized circumstances in your working situation (such as the need to help somebody manage their behaviour) but these are the exception, not the rule. Lead well and honestly when people need you to, but remember that good leading is not about the acquisition of power. If you feel your role as facilitator requires you to 'keep control', reconsider. Try handing over responsibility for key aspects of the group (such as ground rules like punctuality) to members. Give leadership to others in activities. Offer people roles which might otherwise be closed to them, such as learning to operate expensive equipment. Let the group be steered by the aspirations of those who are in it (that includes you).

Product

This can take many forms. Many group members I have worked with have taken away recordings of music created and performed by them. Other groups may work towards a public performance or similarly valued outcome. Your own group's results may be less concrete, but are no less important. Not everything valuable fits into a tape box.

You the facilitator

As someone who has decided to lead music groups, you already possess a unique range of assets. Your *personal creativity* needs to be nurtured and developed; it is what you call upon every time you work. Give yourself room to breathe away from the job. Enjoying music for its own sake is just as important as developing groupwork skills or resources. Whether you sing, play or listen, you will be feeding your musical self. Rest and relax as well; take care of yourself and live creatively.

Your *self-awareness* and *sensitivity to others* are vital assets. It helps enormously to receive positive criticism of your work from someone you trust (this is true even for experienced groupworkers). We all have a lot to learn about ourselves and the ways we relate to others. Be honest with, as well as kind to, yourself. Seek out a mentor for your work.

Your *intent* is another asset. You, and no-one else, decided on your involvement in groupwork. (If this is not so, go back and choose for yourself.) Check your own (not others') expectations of the work you do. Are they positive and open-ended? Expect the best; keep your sense of vision, and do not be put off course by others; you are not responsible for their viewpoint. Remember that positive intent will empower your life and work.

Trust your *intuition*, whether in relation to others or when thinking and acting on your own behalf. It is an internal compass, a tool for planning and an on-the-spot guiding force during the group process.

Finally, remember: *you are your own greatest asset.* Good luck with your groupwork!

SECTION 2

ACTIVITIES

Note: The division into warm-ups, core activities and closures is for ease of reference. Many activities can be used elsewhere in the group process.

REMEMBERING

Resources: Audio or video recording of material from previous session (if available)

■ Activity

1   Spend the first minutes of the group (or a few minutes before a core activity) remembering the previous meeting or a particular activity.

2   Focus on what the group has achieved collectively, as well as any individually memorable moments.

3   Give everyone time to contribute their memories (including your own) and consider playing any relevant audio or video recordings.

PLANNING

Resources: Instruments and equipment (for reference); wallchart
  if required

■ Activity
1   Spend a few minutes early in the group negotiating how the
    present meeting will be used. Give everyone time to contribute
    their ideas (including yourself).
2   Refer, if necessary, to any forward planning decisions made
    previously.

Tip: Any instruments or equipment to be used can be set up first,
as they may be useful in promoting discussion. You can write
people's ideas on a wallchart.

CLAP ROUND

Resources: None

■ Activity
1 Sit in a circle. Each person claps once in turn round the circle.
2 Go round more than once. Speed up after a while. You can reverse the direction of the clapping too.

■ Considerations
1 Some people may find it hard to 'keep the beat', needing support, extra time to clap or a slower pace.
2 If someone cannot clap, do not clap one of their hands with yours unless you alert them first (this can feel like assault).

■ Development
Try more complex clapping activities.

■ Relevant creative/interactive skills
Concentrating; turn-taking.

NAMES AND RHYTHMS

Resources: None

■ Activity

1 Sit in a circle. Focus the group's attention.
2 Ask participants to say their names in turn round the circle. Do this rhythmically, leaving a silent beat in between each name. Try this round a couple of times.
3 Ask each person to fill in the silent beat with one clap (if the person is male) or two (if female). The double claps should be twice as fast so they fill in the silent beat and keep the pulse.
4 Let the whole group clap together after a while.
5 Drop the spoken names, leaving just the claps with silent beats between them. Let the rhythm of the claps become established by letting the group continue for several 'rounds'. Try speeding up.

Tip: Make a joke of it if somebody gets the gender wrong.

■ Considerations

Choose a slower speed and/or vary the rhythmic pulse in order to accommodate people who respond more slowly. You need to hold the focus when doing this.

■ Development

1 Try dividing the group, bringing in the second clappers after a few seconds (cue them positively and precisely). This creates interesting cross-rhythms.
2 Try instruments instead of clapping.
3 Move on to activities like 'Building Rhythms' (page 34) or 'Tribal Chanting' (page 44).

■ Relevant creative/interactive skills

Remembering names; combining rhythms.

NAME RAP

Resources: None

■ Activity
1 Sit in a circle. Ask everyone to say their name once round the group. Repeat this once or twice (especially if it is a new group).
2 Invite people to chant the names they have heard, like this: John and Peter, Peter and Susan, Susan and Bridget (the underlined syllables are the strong beats).
3 Set up a swinging, but not too fast, rhythm with the names. Clap hands, click fingers or slap thighs on the off-beats (the ones not underlined above), like this:

John and Peter, Peter and Susan (etc)

     x   x   x   x (clicks)

4 Speed up.
5 Try more exotic rhythms (it will feel dance-like).

■ Considerations
Some groups can try this more slowly.

■ Development
1 Try other clapping activities.
2 Try 'Building Rhythms' (page 34) or 'Tribal Chanting' (page 44).

■ Relevant creative/interactive skills
Developing the creative impulse; concentrating.

CLAPPING AND STAMPING

Resources: None

■ Activity
1 Sit in a circle. Ask people to stamp once, leaving a silent beat afterwards. Do this round the group.
2 Set it up as a pattern and let everyone join in.
3 Add a clap, finger click or thigh slap on the silent beat.
4 Try claps, clicks and slaps in turn.
5 Speed up.
6 When you stop, ask the group for more rhythm ideas (add half-beats too).

■ Considerations
1 Try a slower or more flexible pace for people with a physical and/or learning disability.
2 Try a three-beat pattern (stamp/clap/clap).

■ Development
Try 'Building Rhythms' (page 34) and 'Tribal Chanting' (page 44).

■ Relevant creative/interactive skills
Establishing (a beat); elaborating; intensifying; concentrating.

OPEN DAY

Resources: Instruments

■ Activity

1 Lay out the instruments as part of the group seating arrangement (I recommend a circle of chairs). Some may be between chairs, others in the centre of the group on the floor or a low table (useful for small instruments if people find it difficult to reach them).

2 Introduce the instruments (perhaps as 'sound sources'). The group may want to check the names of unfamiliar ones. Explain that instruments are valuable and should be treated with respect, but that normal use (including heavy playing) is fine. Tell people (if you have not already done so) that they do not have to be 'skilled' or 'musical' to try them.

3 Offer a period of time for everyone to explore the collection and select an instrument.

4 Encourage people to mingle, experiment and swop.

Tip: The group may wish to help unpack and assemble the instruments at the start of the group. This may need to be supervised.

■ Considerations

1 If anyone has mobility problems or feels inhibited, take or show them some instruments.

2 If choosing is hard, offer two or three from which to select.

■ Development

1 This is a good starting-point for instrumental groupwork.

2 As an exercise in trust and empathy, ask people to choose an instrument for someone else.

■ Relevant creative/interactive skills

Exploring; choosing.

Cautionary note

Cross-infection can occur if a used mouthpiece is passed to another player without being cleaned. *You may already be obliged to follow control of infection rules in your place of work.* Make sure mouthpieces are cleaned and dried before being used again. There are a number of lightly medicated sprays on the market which are good for this purpose.

WHICH ONE'S FOR ME?

Resources: The group does not have to play in this activity, but the instruments should be present

■ **Activity**
1   Sit in a circle. Ask group members which instrument they would choose if they were going to play. Discuss and explore the reasons for their choices.
2   Explain that they can demonstrate their choice by playing an instrument if they wish, but that there is no pressure to do so.

■ **Consideration**
Individuals or whole groups who are unsure about playing may feel more at ease speaking about, rather than trying, instruments.

■ **Development**
1   Ask people which instrument they would *not* choose.
2   Move into playing.

■ **Relevant creative/interactive skills**
Choosing a sound; awareness of own needs; listening and sharing.

PLAYING IN TURN

Resources: Instruments

■ Activity
1 Sit in a circle. Ask individuals to choose an instrument.
2 Suggest they play their chosen instruments in turn. Invite or choose someone to go first. You may suggest that people play only for a short time, or let events take their course.
3 You can suggest players turn and look at the next person as a cue.
4 Group members may want to stop and talk about the experience, interrupting the flow of the activity. You may feel this is reasonable in the early stages of a group, or suggest that people play without comment (the latter usually feels more musical).
5 Speed up the pace and momentum.

Tip: People may stop and laugh at the novelty of the experience. Make this positive for them and the group: it's fun.

■ Consideration
If people 'jump the queue' or play again before their turn arrives, kneel in the centre of the group and use gestural and/or verbal prompts to encourage turn-taking.

■ Development
This activity leads well into 'Conversations', page 29.

■ Relevant creative/interactive skills
Listening and sharing; taking turns.

GUESS THE FEELING

Resources: Instruments

■ **Activity**
1 Sit in a circle. Ask everyone to choose an instrument which sounds like the way they feel today.
2 Play in turn round the circle.
3 When everyone has played (perhaps more than once), ask group members to guess others' feelings. Encourage players to wait for guesses before disclosing their own feelings. You may need to help rephrase guesses if they seem too personal or negative.

■ **Considerations**
1 This activity can be useful for people who find it difficult to verbalize feelings.
2 People may say they feel 'OK' or 'fine' when their playing sounds very different.
3 Let the group choose how far they want to take this activity. There can be quite a jump between talking about a sound and disclosing feelings.

■ **Development**
This is a useful early activity for personal growth or expressive skills work.

■ **Relevant creative/interactive skills**
Choosing a sound; taking turns; awareness of own feelings; listening and sharing.

WHAT'S IT LIKE?

Resources: Instruments

■ Activity

1 Sit in a circle. Ask group members to choose an instrument.
2 Ask everyone to play in turn round the circle.
3 When everyone has played (perhaps more than once), ask them what particular sounds remind them of. A tambourine may sound Spanish or 'like the Salvation Army'; a gong may remind someone of 'the man at the start of old films'. Encourage players to listen to others' thoughts before offering their own.

■ Consideration

This activity can be useful for people who find it difficult to share with others. Feelings are bound to be discussed, but in a less personal way than in 'Guess the Feeling' (page 25).

■ Development

This is a good preparation for 'Programme Improvisation' (page 58) or other depictive work.

■ Relevant creative/interactive skills

Choosing a sound; taking turns; listening and sharing.

GUESS THE CREATURE

Resources: Instruments

■ Activity
1 Sit in a circle. Ask the group to choose instruments that sound like animals.
2 Ask individuals to play in turn round the circle. Listen to, and guess, people's chosen sounds. This can involve the feeling of the sound as well as its more depictive characteristics. Encourage participants to hear all guesses before they disclose their chosen creature.

Tip: The guesses may be more inventive than the answers!

■ Consideration
This activity may be unsuitable for people with mental health problems.

■ Development
1 Try different topics, such as weather.
2 Try this as a vocal activity; move on to 'The Jungle', page 43, 'Sound Pictures 1', page 70 and 'Sound Pictures 2', page 72.
3 Try other depictive activities such as 'Programme Improvisation', page 58, 'Improvising Soundtracks 1', page 60 and 'Improvising Soundtracks 2', page 62.

■ Relevant creative/interactive skills
Choosing a sound; taking turns; painting with sound; listening and sharing.

PASS THE SOUND

Resources: Instruments

■ Activity
1 Sit in a circle. Ask group members to choose an instrument.
2 Ask someone to make up a short sound or simple rhythm, then 'pass it on' round the group. Encourage each player to make eye contact with the next to play. Go round a few times.
3 Try speeding up; change the direction of the turn-taking, or 'bounce' turns around the group unpredictably.

Tip: Do not worry about different types of instruments, as the phrase will change anyway.

■ Consideration
The pace of this activity may need to be slower for some groups, and consecutive turn-taking may be easier at first.

■ Development
1 Try only one type of instrument (eg. blown).
2 Make the sounds longer or the rhythms more complex.

■ Relevant creative/interactive skills
Choosing a sound; listening and sharing; turn-taking.

CONVERSATIONS

Resources: Instruments, particularly swannee whistles (these have an internal mechanism which lets the player 'slide' up and down the whole range of the instrument)

■ Activity
1   Sit in a circle. Introduce the concept of dialogue, stressing the importance of listening. Offer a chance to 'talk and listen, but with no words'.
2   Ask two people to choose an instrument. You may suggest they use swannee whistles, as these are the most fun (they mimic speech well). Ask them to have a chat together using the instruments. You may or may not suggest a time limit — it is often more important to suggest that the chats should not be too short! Encourage the group to listen.
3   Ask the group what the content or subject of the conversation might have been. This could include guessing the moods of the two 'talkers'.
4   Repeat the activity with other participants.

Tip: Do not get bogged down in literal syllabic translations of musical phrases (although some will be amusingly clear!); focusing on feelings conveyed by each player will help move away from this.

■ Considerations
1   Some people may need help to play the swannee whistle.
2   If turn-taking is difficult, try gestural and/or verbal prompts.
3   Some people may need individual support.

■ Development
1   Try three-way conversations.
2   Seat players back-to-back.

■ Relevant creative/interactive skills
Choosing a sound; being spontaneous; listening and sharing.

GAMELAN FOR TWO*

Resources: Metallophone or xylophone, drum, tape recorder (if used)

■ Activity

1 Invite two people to play the same metallophone or xylophone, sitting on opposite sides. The instrument should be tuned to the 'black notes' (pentatonic) scale (see 'Adapting instruments for maximum effectiveness' in Section 3). Suggest they can:

   (a) start by 'talking' to each other on the instrument;
   (b) play freely;
   (c) set up a pulse;
   (d) make up different rhythms together in the pulse;
   (e) get faster;
   (f) decide what the signal will be to finish (if any).

2 Ask the group to listen, then share their impressions.
3 You can record the music and listen to it afterwards.

■ Considerations

Someone with a physical or learning disability may find it difficult to set up a pulse and improvise in it. Free playing is just fine. Try a 'conversation' and let it develop into simultaneous playing.

■ Development

1 Ask a third player to set up a pulse on a drum after the music has started.
2 Try 'Solos and Accompaniments' (pages 49–51) or other rhythmic activities.

■ Relevant creative/interactive skills

Developing the creative impulse; listening and sharing.

*(Gamelan is the Indonesian tuned percussion orchestra. Gamelan music is full of fast, combined phrases.)

30

STOP!

Resources: Instruments, tape recorder (if used)

■ Activity

1   Sit in a half-circle with a 'leader's chair' in the space. Explain that the leader can stop the group by making her own sound. Choose this sound (something played on a loud instrument might seem the obvious choice, but I recommend something quieter, such as a chime bar, wind wand or softly played woodblock).

2   Let the group play freely, quietly at first, then with increasing excitement and volume. The leader has a number of chances to stop the improvisation by playing her own instrument. When she finishes playing, have a moment's silence before the group resumes.

3   You can record the activity and listen to it afterwards.

4   The group can give positive feedback to the leader about how clear the cues were for them, and how much (or little) time they had to play between stops.

■ Consideration

The leader's role can be good for someone who lacks confidence or who is over-impulsive (since there are only a finite number of chances to stop the group).

■ Development

1   The leader can change instruments and/or nominate a successor.

2   Move on to 'Basic Directing Gestures' and associated activities (pages 52–55).

3   Try 'Solos and Accompaniments' (pages 49–51).

■ Relevant creative/interactive skills

Developing the creative impulse; leading; following.

31

HOLD BACK THE TIDE

Resources: Instruments, tape recorder (if used)

■ Activity

1   Sit in a circle. Share with the group the idea that a tide comes in slowly but is unstoppable. Ask them to try and hold back the 'tide of sound' for as long as they can before it rises.

2   Suggest that they listen to the individual waves and ripples of sound ebbing and flowing. After the tide is full, the sound can slowly ebb away.

3   Ask the group to choose 'tidal' instruments (cymbals, gongs, ocean drums, bells and so on).

4   Have a short silence before and after playing.

5   You can record the music and listen to it afterwards.

6   Ask what the group noticed and heard: not just individual sounds, but also the texture and feel of the whole music. It is helpful to encourage people to speak about more than just their own sound. If playing again, the group might try other instruments too.

■ Considerations

1   Some people may find it hard to control their impulse to get louder quickly.

2   Nervous or inhibited people may wish to listen at first.

3   This activity may be unsuitable for people with mental health problems.

■ Development

1   Try 'Programme Improvisation' (page 58).

2   The feelings evoked by the experience can be used in personal growth work.

■ Relevant creative/interactive skills

Choosing a sound; painting with sound; listening and sharing.

TWO GROUPS

Resources: Instruments, tape recorder (if used)

■ Activity

1   Sit participants in two half-circles. Ask each group to choose instruments of contrasting tone colours and/or volume, creating separate 'groups of sound'.
2   Each group improvises in turn. Share the suggestions in 'Free Improvisation' (page 56) before playing. Let each group have three or four turns. You may cue each group or let one take their cue from the other.
3   You can record the improvisation and listen to it together afterwards.
4   After playing, discuss what the different groups of sounds felt or sounded like. It is helpful to encourage people to speak about more than just their own sound.

■ Consideration

This activity is not meant to involve 'battling with sound ' (although this is sometimes fun). If it gets this way, mix loud and quiet instruments in each group and/or mix sexes.

■ Development

1   Try three groups.
2   You can introduce 'Basic Directing Gestures' (page 52) as a focus for group turn-taking and as a way of varying the sounds.
3   Use 'Swop' (page 36).
4   Try two or three groups of players in 'Programme Improvisation' (page 58).

■ Relevant creative/interactive skills

Choosing a sound; developing the creative impulse; listening and sharing; collaborating.

BUILDING RHYTHMS

Resources: Rhythm instruments (clapping may be used instead), other instruments if required, tape recorder (if used)

■ Activity
1 Ask someone to make up a short rhythmic phrase (the simpler the better). Add other players.
2 Stop. Ask for a second pattern at the same speed and pulse (one strong beat in every four, or every three, etc). Add other players.
3 Stop. Restart the first pattern, cueing in the second after a moment (be positive and precise).
4 Let both rhythms run together. Add additional parts one by one. These do not have to start on the first (strong) beat of the pulse; it is more exciting if off-beats and even half-beats appear. Introduce other colours, such as cymbals and gongs.
5 Cue the finish by beat or gesture.
6 Swop instruments and rhythms when repeating.
7 You can record the music and listen to it afterwards.

Tip: Have some example rhythms ready to start this activity and be ready to demonstrate, perhaps by adding the second rhythm yourself, at first.

■ Considerations
1 Try slower speeds and/or simpler patterns for the first two parts.
2 Try unusual sounds like 'rolled' cymbals or gongs over the top of the rhythms.
3 Ask someone to cue the finish.

■ Development
1 If you start by clapping, move to instruments.
2 Experiment with more complex rhythms and different pulses (eg. simultaneous four- and three-beat patterns).
3 Use tuned percussion (choose pitches that sound well together: see 'Adapting instruments for maximum effectiveness' in Section 3).
4 Try becoming louder or (especially) softer, as well as faster.
5 Move on to 'Solos and Accompaniments' (pages 49–51).

■ Relevant creative/interactive skills

Developing the creative impulse; sharing and listening; concentrating; leading and following.

SWOP

Resources: Instruments from current activity

■ Activity

Use this idea when it feels right to swop instruments. Invite people to
change their instrument for another. You can:

   (a)   say that instruments have to be passed on if other
   people ask for them;

   (b)   alternatively, ask everyone to hand their instrument to
   the person on the right (or the left).

Tip: Mediate if you need to (some instruments are very popular).

■ Consideration

Some people may need help to move larger instruments.

■ Development

Try passing all the players' instruments right round the circle so that
everyone can play them in turn (see cautionary note on page 21).

■ Relevant creative/interactive skills

Sharing.

SCRATCH ARRANGEMENTS

Resources: See 'Arranging music from scratch' in Section 3 for help in preparing this activity: you need to prepare the instruments specified in the arrangement; tape recorder (if used)

■ Activity
1   Sit in a half-circle with you in the space. Organize players with their instruments. If your arrangement is new to the group, ask people to guess what it is from hearing a few notes.
2   All play (and sing) it through. (You need to direct the activity — see 'Developing skills of direction' in Section 3).
3   Let people swop or take over parts in the arrangement.
4   You can record the music and listen to it afterwards.

Tip: Playing scratch arrangements should be fun, rather than stressful — do not be a maestro at the expense of enjoyment.

■ Considerations
1   Design or adapt parts beforehand to suit the abilities of individual players.
2   Be aware of group members who need extra time to play, or to master a more complex part. Try the activity over slowly, pausing when necessary; with practice you will retain musical cohesion (a confident singing voice helps here).
3   Taking over the director's role is good for someone who lacks confidence.

■ Development
1   Have several ideas for arrangements 'up your sleeve', as they make good warm-ups for many groups.
2   Try more complex arrangements.
3   Ask people to choose what music they want to play.
4   Let others direct.

■ Relevant creative/interactive skills
Concentrating; leading and following.

BREATHING A SOUND

Resources: None

■ Activity
1 Darken the room.
2 Stand in a circle. Participants may want to close their eyes.
3 Ask them to breathe slowly in and out, guided by your voice. Use a slow count of three for the in-breath and another for the exhalation.
4 After a few moments, ask people to notice what their breathing feels like. Guide their attention to their throat, shoulders, torso and stomach in turn as they continue to breathe. Suggest they have a 'channel of air' opening and flowing through their bodies. You will probably not need to count any more.
5 Ask people to notice the sound of their breathing. Suggest that, when they exhale, they can let their breath turn into any sound that it chooses. Ask them not to think about the pitch or musical quality of the sound, just how it feels for them. Encourage them to let go and enjoy the experience.
6 When you have finished, have a few moments' silence, then ask group members to open their eyes when they feel comfortable. You can leave the lights low for a while.
7 Ask the group to share their experiences of vocalizing.

Tip: Some people may want to listen at first.

■ Considerations
1 This activity may be unsuitable for people with mental health problems.
2 Some people may find the experience disturbing.
3 Suggest people sit or lie down if they feel faint or dizzy.

■ Development
1 Use the activity as a start to vocal improvisation work.
2 Use as part of personal growth work.
3 Use as a closing group activity.

■ Relevant creative/interactive skills
Self-awareness; creating a sound.

TONING

Resources: None

■ Activity

1   Darken or black out the room.
2   Stand in a circle. Suggest people close their eyes.
3   You could preface this activity with 'Breathing a Sound' (page 38). Ask the group to start humming quietly on a comfortably low-pitched note. Explain that you will set a note to start, but people can hum at whatever pitch comes naturally to them. Remind them to breathe! The sound should be continuous, ebbing and flowing freely.
4   After a while, ask the group to listen and join you in making some vowel sounds. Try moving through 'ah', 'eh', 'ee', 'oh' and 'oo', changing the shape of the mouth slowly to make a smooth transition. Take your time. Encourage people to let go and enjoy the sound.
5   When you have finished, have a short silence, then ask participants to open their eyes when they feel comfortable. You might leave the lights low for a while.
6   Ask the group to share their experiences of vocalizing.

Tip: Some people may just want to listen at first.

■ Considerations

1   This activity may be unsuitable for people with mental health problems.
2   Some people may find the experience disturbing.
3   Suggest people sit or lie down if they feel faint or dizzy.

■ Development

1   Use the activity as a start to vocal improvisation work.
2   Use as part of personal growth work.
3   Use as a closing group activity.

■ Relevant creative/interactive skills

Self-awareness; creating and transforming sounds.

OVERTONING

Resources: None

■ Activity

1 Darken or black out the room.
2 Stand in a circle. Suggest people close their eyes.
3 You could preface this activity with 'Breathing a Sound' (page 38). Ask the group to start humming quietly on a comfortably low-pitched note. Explain that you will a set a note to start, but people can hum at whatever pitch comes naturally to them. Remind them to breathe! The sound should be continuous, ebbing and flowing freely.
4 After a while, ask the group to focus their voice in the front portion of the mouth, just behind the front teeth. Draw their attention to the rich overtones in the sound as you cycle slowly through the vowels 'ah', 'eh', 'ee', 'oh' and 'oo'. Encourage people to let go and enjoy the sound.
5 When you have finished, have a short silence, then ask participants to open their eyes when they feel comfortable. You might leave the lights low for a while.
6 Ask the group to share their experiences of vocalizing.

Tip: Some people may just want to listen at first.

■ Considerations

1 This activity may be unsuitable for people with mental health problems.
2 Some people may find the experience disturbing.
3 Suggest people sit or lie down if they feel faint or dizzy.

■ Development

1 Use the activity as a start to vocal improvisation work.
2 Use as part of personal growth work.
3 Use as a closing group activity.

■ Relevant creative/interactive skills

Self-awareness; creating and transforming sounds.

BOUNCE

Resources: None

■ Activity
1 Darken or black out the room.
2 Sit in a circle. You could ask people to close their eyes.
3 Ask group members to make up short/sharp/surprising (but not necessarily loud) vocal sounds . Ask the group to listen for and respond to others' sounds, 'bouncing' them round the group.
4 People can share their impressions afterwards.

Tip: Some people may just want to listen at first.

■ Development
1 Try voices and instruments together.
2 Try an instrumental sound and a vocal response, or vice versa.
3 Move on to 'Mountain Tribes' (page 42) or 'The Jungle' (page 43).
4 Try 'Mouth Music' (page 74).

■ Relevant creative/interactive skills
Choosing a sound; being spontaneous; listening and sharing.

MOUNTAIN TRIBES

Resources: None (unless instruments are used); a very large room is useful

■ Activity
1 It helps if the room is dim. Ask the group to split into two, and to go as far into separate corners of the room as possible.
2 Explain that, like people on distant mountains, they can communicate by sound, not words.
3 The two groups can call wordlessly to each other, listening for the others' reply. It helps if single people do this first and others then join in. Try yodelling, ululating and so on. Ask participants to listen to the calls and answer them. The calls can grow in intensity and complexity, overlap and combine.
4 When they have finished, the groups can join together and discuss the experience. Ask people to guess the feelings and content of the other group's calls.

Tip: Some people may listen first and take part later.

■ Development
1 Try voices and instruments.
2 Try this in two different rooms with the doors open between them (check who is around!).
3 Try 'The Jungle' (page 43) and other vocal activities.
4 Try using three tribes.

■ Relevant creative/interactive skills
Choosing a sound; being spontaneous; developing the creative impulse; translating experience into sound; listening and sharing; collaborating.

THE JUNGLE

Resources: Tape recorder (if used)

■ Activity
1 Darken or black out the room.
2 Sit in a circle. Ask the group to close their eyes. Ask them to imagine they are in a jungle, teeming with life of all kinds. They can create the atmosphere vocally in any way they wish. Some possibilities:

   (a) creature sounds (birds, animals, insects);
   (b) water or wind sounds;
   (c) trees bending, branches cracking and so on.

3 Suggest that:

   (a) people can listen and respond to someone else's sound (rather than vocalize continuously);
   (b) people can listen to the group as a whole;
   (c) the sounds will ebb and flow, and it is fine just to stop and listen;
   (d) there will be a silence first, and you will start if no-one else does.

4 Hold the silence for a short while at the end of the improvisation.
5 You can record the sounds and listen to them afterwards.
6 Ask the group to share their experience. Ask what they noticed and heard, not just individual sounds, but also the way in which the atmosphere built up. It is helpful to encourage people to speak about more than just their own sound.

Tip: Some people may just want to listen at first.

■ Development
1 Try whistling, body sounds and so on.
2 Move on to 'Sound Pictures 1' (page 70) and 'Sound Pictures 2'' (page 72).

■ Relevant creative/interactive skills
Choosing a sound; painting with sound; listening and sharing.

TRIBAL CHANTING

Resources: Drums (a wide selection is useful)

■ Activity

1   Sit in a circle. Ask group members to choose a hand-played drum.
2   Darken the room (if it is blacked out, people will not see to play). Improvise on drums together. Try setting a common pulse that is compelling rather than fast.
3   After a few moments, invite people to chant or sing wordlessly while they play.
4   Build up the intensity of the drumming and vocalizing. Finish with a pre-arranged signal (gesture or drum beat).
5   Discuss the experience.

Tip: Increasing intensity need not mean increasing speed (although this can be fun).

■ Consideration

Some people may prefer to listen, or just drum, at first.

■ Development

1   Try stopping and restarting the drumming several times while the chanting continues.
2   Ask someone to chant a phrase for everyone to answer. Take turns with this while the drumming continues.
3   Try stopping the drumming while someone chants on their own, then restarting.

■ Relevant creative/interactive skills

Developing the creative impulse; listening and sharing.

WELL-KNOWN SONGS

Resources: A keyboard is useful

■ Activity

It helps to sit in a circle. Ask people what songs they would like to sing, and encourage the group to do this together.

Tip: A community songbook and/or a hymnbook can be useful.

■ Considerations

1   Elderly people often enjoy singing familiar songs together; hymns may also be requested.
2   People with a learning disability are often used to singing age-inappropriate songs in service settings; consider carefully before trying this activity, and be sensitive to their status as adults.

■ Development

Try other vocal activities.

■ Relevant creative/interactive skills

Listening and sharing.

LISTENING TASTES

Resources: Recorded music and listening equipment (a remote control is useful)

■ Activity
1   It helps to sit in a circle. Share and discuss musical tastes (especially if it is a new group).
2   Play a piece of music that you or someone else has brought. After listening, ask the group to share any opinions, impressions or other experiences (for example, evoked memories).
3   Play several pieces if you have time.

Tip: Do not listen to a whole piece if it is too long. Fade it out gently; a sudden stop can be shocking.

■ Considerations
1   Some people can find it difficult to move away from circular 'I like it because it's good' statements. Encourage them to expand on their opinions. You might look first at concrete aspects of the music (speed, volume, singer and so on), then at the impressions or atmosphere evoked.
2   Some people may feel they will cause offence if they offer a negative opinion. Encourage this in the same way, but be sensitive to people who might feel hurt by another's viewpoint.

■ Development
1   This activity can run for several sessions if people bring their own music.
2   If you plan to work on 'TV/Film Tastes' (page 75), 'Hollywood Panel' (page 77) or want to use listening in other ways, this is a useful starter activity.

■ Relevant creative/interactive skills
Listening and sharing (in both the musical and verbal sense); choosing (one's own music).

WARM-UP: LISTENING

QUIZ

Resources: Recorded music (you need a tape recorder and so on as well) or keyboard if you are doing this 'live'; lots of ideas for questions; wallchart scoreboard, if used

■ Activity

1   Sit in a circle or two half-circles, depending on whether it is an individual or group quiz.

2   Your quiz may be any style you choose: informal (to encourage participation) or scored (in which case you will have winners and losers, and need a scorekeeper). Prepare your material in advance. Some ideas:

    (a) pop music (contemporary or 'oldies', including 1940s, etc);

    (b) TV or radio themes (present or past);

    (c) hymns;

    (d) national anthems and songs;

    (e) classical favourites;

    (f) types of music associated with particular dances;

    (g) sound effects;

    (h) music or sound played backwards (see 'Using recording and multitrack equipment' in Section 3);

    (i) 'Name that tune in three notes (or four, five, etc)'.

    (j) Winslow's *Musical Quiz* contains 80 pre-recorded melodies that are ideal for this type of activity.

Since every quiz idea has been used by broadcasters at some time, there is no lack of choice.

Tip: If you play keyboard well (especially if you can play by ear) it makes a quiz more fun than when using recorded music.

■ Considerations

1   If someone cannot answer easily, offer a choice of answers. Consider signed or pointed responses as an option.

2   If one group member 'gets in first' all the time, offer questions to individuals rather than everyone.

47

3 You can lead this activity quite firmly without causing rancour, as most people are used to quizmasters on television.

■ Development
Let someone else be quizmaster.

■ Relevant creative/interactive skills
Problem-solving; listening and sharing.

SOLOS AND ACCOMPANIMENTS 1

Resources: Instruments, tape recorder (if used)

■ Activity
1   Sit in a circle. Ask for two players.
2   Give one player a metallophone with two identified low-pitched bars tuned a fifth apart, and two beaters. The pitch of the bars should not be so low as to lack the 'resonance' of a perfect fifth (see 'Adapting instruments for maximum effectiveness' in Section 3). Ask the other player to choose a 'solo' instrument. Suggestions: melodica (a reed instrument with piano style keys; try playing just the white ones here), swannee whistle, harmonica, talking drum (varies in pitch) or xylophone (pentatonic tuning — see Section 3).
3   The metallophone player sounds the bars in a 'tremolo' (notes repeated freely and fairly fast). The other player waits for a few moments before creating a free 'solo' above this background. The metallophone player waits for the end of the solo before finishing.
4   You can record the music and listen to it afterwards.
5   Ask others to listen and share impressions. Ask the players how it felt to 'solo' and support.

■ Considerations
1   A tremolo texture for tuned percussion can be split between two people if two-handed playing is difficult.
2   Some people can find prolonged tremolo playing tiring.

■ Development
1   The supporting texture can be created by several people playing instruments freely. Some suggestions: chime bars (selected pitches), metallophone (selected bars), keyboard, xylophone (selected bars), bell ropes and sprays (these are hand-held 'jingles') and/or wind wands (flexible tubes that 'sing' high notes when whirled around). See also next activity.
2   Several soloists on different instruments can take turns.
3   This activity can form part of a larger-scale piece.
4   Try a wordless vocal solo with instrumental accompaniment.

■ Relevant creative/interactive skills
Choosing a sound; developing the creative impulse; listening and sharing; supporting.

CORE ACTIVITY: INSTRUMENTAL

SOLOS AND ACCOMPANIMENTS 2

Resources: Instruments, tape recorder (if used)

■ Activity
1 See previous activity. In this version the 'free' accompaniment is replaced by an ostinato (regular rhythm) texture.
2 Ask for two or more 'supporters' and offer a selection of instruments. Some suggestions:

    (a) chime bars (selected pitches);
    (b) metallophone or xylophone (selected bars);
    (c) keyboard;
    (d) rhythm instruments.

3 Follow the process in 'Building Rhythms' (page 34) to create and combine at least two repeated short phrases and/or rhythms, then add others if appropriate. This will take a little time.
4 You can add other freely played instruments like bell ropes/sprays or wind wand (see page 49).
5 The chosen soloist improvises above the supporting texture. The solo can be influenced by the rhythmic patterns of the accompaniment, or flow above them.
6 You can record the music and listen to it afterwards.
7 Ask the rest of the group to listen and share impressions . Ask the players how it felt to 'solo' and support.

Tip: Do not have too complex a texture.

■ Considerations
See 'Building Rhythms' (page 34).

■ Development
1 Several soloists on different instruments can take turns.
2 This activity can form part of a larger-scale piece.
3 Try a wordless vocal solo with instrumental accompaniment.

■ Relevant creative/interactive skills
Choosing a sound; developing the creative impulse; purposefulness; listening and sharing; supporting.

BASIC DIRECTING GESTURES

Resources: None

■ Activity

Demonstrate, and ask the group to copy, the following gestures, which will be used in 'Directing 1' (page 53), 'Directing 2' (page 54) and 'Directing 3' (page 55).

1 Play: extend your arm and hand.
2 Stop: like a policeman, with upraised hand.
3 Louder: raise extended arm.
4 Softer: lower extended arm *and/or* put finger to mouth.
5 Faster: quickening circular hand movements.
6 Slower: slowing circular hand movements.
7 Cueing several players: a horizontal movement of the extended arm to include players seated next to each other *or* successive brief gestures to players seated apart.
8 Continue playing: a circular hand movement, distinguished from (**5**) and (**6**) by being shorter.

DIRECTING 1

Resources: Instruments, video camera and TV (if used)

■ Activity

1 The group sits in a half-circle. Explain that this is an opportunity for someone to take charge of the sounds being made. Say that this can be done without any words. Explain that this kind of directing does not mean beating time, just letting people know how you want them to play.
2 Introduce directing gestures (**1**) to (**6**) (see page 52).
3 Ask one player to choose a rhythm or tuned percussion instrument. Invite a volunteer to take charge of the created sound. The director can stand or sit in front of the group.
4 Director and player create a short piece. Ask the group to watch and listen.
5 You can video the activity and watch it afterwards.
6 The group can share their impressions afterwards and give positive feedback to both people.

Tip: Most people do not use clear or large enough gestures when they first try this.

■ Considerations

1 People who lack confidence or who have poor body awareness can benefit from the experience of directing.
2 Physically disabled people and those with a disorder of communication may need support.
3 Some players can find it hard to concentrate on the director's gestures.
4 Visually impaired players will need support.

■ Development

See 'Directing 2' (page 54) and 'Directing 3' (page 55).

■ Relevant creative/interactive skills

Developing the creative impulse; listening and sharing; leading and following.

DIRECTING 2

Resources: Instruments, video camera and TV (if used)

■ Activity
1   Refer to 'Directing 1' (page 53). This is an opportunity for two or three people, and eventually the whole group, to be directed.
2   Gestures (**1**) to (**8**) are needed (see page 52).
3   The group allows the director complete freedom to 'mould' the sound.
4   You can video the activity and watch it afterwards.

Tip: Most people are unsure of their ability to keep several sounds 'in the air' simultaneously, and may prefer to cue and stop players sequentially at first.

■ Considerations
See 'Directing 1' (page 53).

■ Development
1   Try vocal sounds.
2   Try 'Directing 3' (page 55).
3   Try 'Directing Soundtracks' (page 63), 'Stories' (page 64), 'Composing with Wallscore 1' (page 65) and 'Composing with Wallscore 2' (page 66).

■ Relevant creative/interactive skills
Developing the creative impulse; concentrating; listening and sharing; leading and following.

DIRECTING 3

Resources: Instruments, video camera and TV (if used)

■ Activity

1   Refer to 'Directing 1' (page 53) and 'Directing 2' (page 54). Gestures (**1**) to (**8**) are needed (see page 52).

2   Ask people to split into two or three groups and choose similar-sounding instruments in each group (you will need to have enough people for this to work well). Choosing the instruments may take a little time.

3   The director then cues 'groups of sounds' instead of individual players, rather like the sections of an orchestra.

4   You can video the activity and watch it afterwards.

■ Considerations

See 'Directing 1' (page 53).

■ Development

1   Try vocal sounds.

2   Try 'Directing Soundtracks' (page 63), 'Stories' (page 64), 'Composing with Wallscore 1' (page 65) and 'Composing with Wallscore 2' (page 66).

■ Activity

Choosing sounds; developing the creative impulse; listening and sharing; leading and following; collaborating.

CORE ACTIVITY: INSTRUMENTAL

FREE IMPROVISATION

Resources: Instruments, tape recorder (if used)

■ **Activity**
1 Sit in a circle. Ask group members to choose an instrument.
2 Explain that this is a chance to make sound freely. Suggest that:

   (a) participants can listen and respond to someone else's sound (rather than play continuously);
   (b) they can listen to the group as a whole;
   (c) there will probably be no beat or pulse;
   (d) the sounds will ebb and flow, and it is fine just to stop and listen;
   (e) there will be a silence first, and you will start if no-one else does.

3 Let the improvisation happen in its own time. Have a moment's silence afterwards.
4 You can record the improvisation and play it back afterwards.
5 After playing, encourage the group to share their experiences. Ask what they noticed and heard, not just individual sounds, but also the texture and feel of the whole music. It is helpful to encourage people to speak about more than just their own sound.

Tip: Tell everyone, when playing, to release their minds and go with the flow.

■ **Considerations**
1 People who are nervous or inhibited may wish to sit out and listen.
2 Some people may find such an unstructured and spontaneous activity difficult to cope with.
3 This activity may be unsuitable for people with mental health problems.

■ Development
Free improvisation is a core concept in music groupwork. It is central to 'Improvising for Personal Growth 1' (page 67) and 'Improvising for Personal Growth 2' (page 69) as well as many other activities in this manual, and is a useful process for group composing.

■ Relevant creative/interactive skills
Choosing a sound; developing the creative impulse; listening and sharing.

PROGRAMME IMPROVISATION

Resources: Instruments, tape recorder (if used)

■ Activity

1   Sit in a circle. Introduce the concept of 'painting a picture with sound'. Ask the group for ideas. Some suggestions:

   (a) types of weather (rain, snow, wind);
   (b) natural features (a river, the sea, the desert, high mountains);
   (c) places with special characteristics (an old abandoned house, a busy street);
   (d) events (a battle, firework display or football match).

2   Before playing, think together about the characteristics of the idea that has been chosen. A river may be flowing and peaceful, or a noisy torrent. An abandoned house may be eerie and full of echoes. Be imaginative about the sonic possibilities, as well as the feelings or atmosphere evoked by the idea.

3   Ask the group to choose instruments that will evoke the sounds and feelings of their idea. Suggest they keep their chosen idea as a 'mental picture' while they play. Start and finish with a short silence.

4   You can record the improvisation and listen to it afterwards.

5   After playing, encourage the group to share their impressions. Ask what they noticed and heard, not just individual sounds, but also the texture and feel of the whole music. It is helpful to encourage people to speak about more than just their own sound.

6   If playing again, the group may decide to select different instruments.

■ Considerations

1   The process of discussing ideas and choosing sounds may need to be longer in some groups.

2   People who are nervous or inhibited will probably find this activity more accessible than 'Free Improvisation' (page 56) although you will still need to be sensitive about working with the feelings evoked by the process.

3 This activity may be unsuitable for people with mental health problems.

___

■ Development
1 Try 'Improvising Soundtracks 1' (page 60), 'Improvising Soundtracks 2' (page 62), 'Directing Soundtracks' (page 63) and 'Stories' (page 64).
2 The feelings evoked by the programme can also be used in personal growth work.

___

■ Relevant creative/interactive skills
Choosing a sound; painting with sound; listening and sharing.

IMPROVISING SOUNDTRACKS 1

Resources: Instruments, video material, player and TV *or* slides, slide projector and screen; wallchart, tape recorder

■ Activity

1   Prepare video material beforehand (see 'Using video resources' in Section 3) . The sequences can be fairly short, lasting perhaps 4 or 5 minutes. If using slides, choose them beforehand and check they are in order in the projector cartridge.

2   Sit in a half-circle facing the TV or screen. Watch the material together (if the video has a soundtrack, turn it off) and discuss both the concrete (eg. what is on the screen) and evoked elements. The 'missing sounds' can be guessed. You can write key descriptive words on a wallchart.

3   Ask the group to choose instruments with their ideas in mind.

4   Improvise together while the video or slides are shown once more. Ask group members to watch the images and respond to them.

5   Record the music and play it back with the images afterwards.

6   Ask the group about their soundtrack; for example:

   (a)   Did the music feel right?

   (b)   Was it loud/soft/fast/slow/varied enough?

   (c)   Did it have the appropriate atmosphere?

   (d)   Did particular sounds match particular images or events?

   (e)   What instruments felt appropriate (ie what can be changed)?

   (f)   Were there too many sounds at once?

   (g)   Is a director needed? (see 'Directing Soundtracks', page 63).

7   The group might rerecord after deciding any changes.

Tip: You will probably need to delegate the operation of some of the equipment.

■ Considerations

1   See 'Programme Improvisation' (page 58).

2   Visually impaired people will need to be told about the images.

3 People with a learning disability and/or a disorder of communication may find it difficult to create sounds for more abstract images.

4 Nervous or inhibited people may prefer 'Hollywood Panel' (page 77).

■ Development
Try 'Improvising Soundtracks 2' (page 62), 'Directing Soundtracks' (page 63) and 'Stories' (page 64).

■ Relevant creative/interactive skills
Choosing a sound; developing the creative impulse; painting with sound; listening and sharing.

IMPROVISING SOUNDTRACKS 2

Resources: Instruments, video material, player and TV *or* slides, slide projector and screen; wallchart, tape recorder

■ Activity
1   See previous activity.
2   Try vocal improvisation, or a mixture of vocal and instrumental sounds.
3   Record a longer soundtrack, or several sections of music for a sequential piece of video.
4   Make original artwork slides, or shoot an original video.

■ Considerations
1   See 'Programme Improvisation' (page 58).
2   Visually impaired people will need to be told about the images.
3   People with a learning disability and/or a disorder of communication may find it difficult to create sounds for more abstract images.
4   Nervous or inhibited people may prefer 'Hollywood Panel' (page 77).

■ Development
1   Present the final result as a finished piece.
2   Try 'Hollywood Panel' (see page 77).

■ Relevant creative/interactive skills
Choosing a sound; developing the creative impulse; painting with sound; listening and sharing.

CORE ACTIVITY: INSTRUMENTAL

DIRECTING SOUNDTRACKS

Resources: Instruments, video material, player and TV *or* slides, slide projector and screen; wallchart, tape recorder

■ Activity
1   See 'Improvising Soundtracks 1' (page 60) and 'Improvising Soundtracks 2' (page 62).
2   Directing gestures (**1**) – (**8**) are needed (see page 52).
3   Instead of improvising freely, ask for a volunteer to direct the group.

■ Considerations
See 'Directing 1' (page 53) and 'Improvising Soundtracks 2' (page 62).

■ Development
Try 'Stories' (page 64).

■ Relevant creative/interactive skills
Choosing a sound; developing the creative impulse; painting with sound; listening and sharing; leading and following.

STORIES

Resources: Instruments, wallchart (if used), tape recorder (if used)

■ Activity
1 'Programme Improvisation' (page 58) is a good preparation for this activity.
2 Discuss and write up ideas for short 'stories in music': a wallchart is useful. Good ideas should expand around three sections (scene-setting, development and conclusion). Use the process of 'Programme Improvisation' to decide on the sounds for the different parts of the story.
3 Improvise, listen and discuss, as in 'Programme Improvisation'. (This may take more than one session.)

■ Considerations
The process of developing ideas and choosing sounds may need to be longer in some groups.

■ Development
1 Try directing the story; see 'Basic Directing Gestures' (page 52), 'Directing 2' (page 54) and 'Directing 3' (page 55).
2 Write a script for the story and choose a narrator.
3 Try voices instead, or a mixture of voices and instruments.
4 Try 'Composing with Wallscore 1' (page 65) and 'Composing with Wallscore 2' (page 66).

■ Relevant creative/interactive skills
Planning; choosing a sound; painting with sound; listening and sharing.

COMPOSING WITH WALLSCORE 1

Resources: Instruments, wallchart and different coloured pens, tape recorder (if used)

■ Activity

1 Discuss the concept of writing down music. It can be interesting to look at an orchestral score.
2 Ask the group to choose a varied selection of instruments.
3 Invite group members to play their instruments and draw their impression of their sound on the wallchart. Discuss the pictograms and their relationship to the sounds.
4 Separate the pictograms by drawing lines around them, and ask someone to direct a short improvisation by pointing to the drawings as cues for the players. More than one instrument can play at once. Basic directing gestures are useful (see page 52).
5 You can record the music and listen to it afterwards.

■ Considerations

1 See 'Directing 1' (page 53).
2 The pictograms may be hard for some people to see if they are not large enough.

■ Development

Try drawing different kinds of sounds (sharp, flowing, up and down, changing volume or speed, etc).

■ Relevant creative/interactive skills

Choosing a sound; depicting a sound in pictorial form; listening and sharing; leading and following; collaborating.

CORE ACTIVITY: INSTRUMENTAL

COMPOSING WITH WALLSCORE 2

Resources: Instruments, wallchart and different coloured pens, tape recorder (if used)

■ Activity
1 This is a development of the previous activity.
2 Ask the group to choose a varied selection of instruments.
3 Offer the group a chance to 'score their sounds' on the wallchart. Invite people to play their instruments and draw their impression of their sound on the chart, using a horizontal axis from left to right as the 'music line'. Discuss the emerging composition as it develops.
4 Ask someone to direct the written music. Basic directing gestures are useful (see page 52).
5 You can record the music and listen to it afterwards. After listening, the group may want to change the order of musical events or the sounds.

■ Considerations
See 'Directing 1' (page 53).

■ Development
1 Try scoring different kinds of sounds (sharp, flowing, up and down, changing volume or speed, etc).
2 Try more than one line at a time for increasingly complex textures.
3 Try scoring for whole groups of instruments.

NB: This is *not* a way of writing rhythmically barred music, although some groups will be able to do this easily. The written line can include notated events such as sudden starts, stops or sounds, but most people find the mental discipline of 'counting the bars' off-putting and uncreative.

■ Relevant creative/interactive skills
Choosing a sound; depicting a sound in visual form; listening and sharing; leading and following; collaborating.

CORE ACTIVITY: INSTRUMENTAL

IMPROVISING FOR PERSONAL GROWTH 1

Resources: Instruments

■ Activity

Using the following ideas will depend upon the needs of the individuals, and the dynamic of the group, concerned. Your choice will depend on your skill in reading/intuiting others' needs, as well as your previous experience and training.

1 Sit in a circle with the instruments. Before playing, offer suggestions such as the following:

(a) the created sounds may have a feeling or mood;

(b) you may be aware of your own feeling or mood when playing;

(c) the sounds may paint a picture, tell a story, or have a message that you can put into words;

(d) you may like, or dislike, the sounds;

(e) the sounds may remind you of someone;

(f) the sounds may remind you of something about your past or present, or something you anticipate in the future;

(g) you can listen and respond to someone else's sound;

(h) you may be aware of the whole group's sound;

(i) the sounds will ebb and flow, and it is fine just to stop and listen.

2 Be clear about the way you are going to use the improvisation: for example, whether it will be followed by a period of sharing and/or personal exploration, or whether it will stand alone.

3 You can record improvisations and play them back afterwards.

4 Remember to warm up before and wind down after work. See 'Recorded music' in Section 5 for ideas about this.

■ Considerations

1 Psychotherapeutic work may be unsuitable for individuals with mental health problems; if in doubt, seek the guidance of a professional practitioner.

2 People with a learning disability and/or a disorder of communication can also find it difficult to work psychotherapeutically.

■ Development

1 Try vocal work or a mixture of voices and instruments (remember that vocal work can be especially challenging in the context of personal growth work).

2 Consider joint work with a trained psychotherapist.

■ Relevant creative/interactive skills

Confidence to explore and express; developing the creative impulse; translating experience into sound; awareness of own needs; listening and sharing.

IMPROVISING FOR PERSONAL GROWTH 2

Resources: Instruments

■ Activity
1 See previous activity.
2 Here are some other ideas for improvisation on specific topics:

(a) my portrait of myself;
(b) my real feelings;
(c) my hidden feelings;
(d) my forbidden feelings;
(e) my parent/partner/child/boss and myself (with one other player);
(f) my family (with other players).

3 Other ideas will be specific to work in progress.

■ Considerations
1 Psychotherapeutic work may be unsuitable for individuals with mental health problems; if in doubt, seek the guidance of a professional practitioner.
2 People with a learning disability and/or a disorder of communication can also find it difficult to work psychotherapeutically.

■ Development
1 Try vocal work or a mixture of voices and instruments (remember that vocal work can be especially challenging in the context of personal growth work).
2 Consider joint work with a trained psychotherapist.

■ Relevant creative/interactive skills
Confidence to explore and express; developing the creative impulse; translating experience into sound; awareness of own needs; listening and sharing.

SOUND PICTURES 1

Resources: Tape recorder (if used), wallchart (if used)

■ Activity

1   Sit in a circle. Explain that this is a chance to create a 'picture' of a place or event using people's voices. Ask about places or events which have particular sounds associated with them. Examples:

   (a) Thunderstorm: wind, rain, crashing thunder;
   (b) Haunted house: creaky door, footsteps, screams, moans;
   (c) Seaside: gentle surf, bigger waves, seagulls;
   (d) Fairground: rides, yells, stallholders' calls;
   (e) Fireworks display: rockets, bangers, Catherine wheels.

2   You can write ideas on a wallchart.
3   Choose an idea. Darken or black out the room. Ask participants to close their eyes. Suggest that:

   (a) they can listen and respond to someone else's sound (rather than vocalize continuously);
   (b) they can listen to the group as a whole;
   (c) the sounds will ebb and flow, and it is fine just to stop and listen;
   (d) there will be a silence first, and you will start if no-one else does.

4   Hold the silence for a short while at the end of the improvisation.
5   You can record the sound picture and listen to it afterwards.
6   Ask the group to share their impressions. Ask what they noticed and heard, not just individual sounds, but also the ways in which the atmosphere of the picture was built up. It is helpful to encourage people to speak about more than just their own sound.

Tip: Some people may prefer to listen first and take part later.

■ Consideration
This activity may be unsuitable for people with mental health problems.

■ Development
Try 'Sound Pictures 2' (page 72).

■ Relevant creative/interactive skills
Choosing a sound; painting with sound; listening and sharing; collaborating.

SOUND PICTURES 2

Resources: Tape recorder (if used)

■ Activity
1   See 'Sound Pictures 1' (page 70).
2   Participants split into small groups, plan separate sound pictures, then perform them to the group as a whole. They guess others' ideas.

■ Consideration
This activity may be unsuitable for people with mental health problems.

■ Development
1   Try 'body sounds' too (clapping, rubbing hands together, stamping, etc).
2   Try instruments too.
3   Try other programme improvisation activities, using voices instead of instruments.

■ Relevant creative/interactive skills
Choosing a sound; painting with sound; listening and sharing; collaborating.

CORE ACTIVITY: VOCAL

THE SHAMAN

Resources: None

■ Activity
1 Sit in a circle; darken or black out the room.
2 Ask group members to close their eyes.
3 Ask for a volunteer to be the shaman (you might do this at first).
4 Ask the group to hum quietly on a comfortably low-pitched note (set by you, if you wish). After the humming is established, suggest it can change into any open vowel sound that people want to try. Remind them to breathe! The sound will be continuous, ebbing and flowing freely. See 'Toning' (page 39) for more ideas.
5 While the humming continues, the shaman sings or chants a short melodic phrase (no words are needed) repeating it a few times to set the mood. He or she walks slowly round the group, putting a gentle hand on one person's shoulder and singing the phrase to them. The person sings or chants a short answering phrase, and the shaman moves on. The pace should be slow and thoughtful.
6 The shaman ends the activity by gently stamping on the floor (or in some other prearranged way). The other voices can fade out slowly.
7 Hold the silence for a moment afterwards. You might leave the lights low for a while after people have opened their eyes.

■ Considerations
1 If someone wishes not to join in, they can touch the shaman's hand to signify this.
2 This activity may be unsuitable for people with mental health problems.

■ Development
1 People can continue to sing or chant melodically once visited by the shaman, the whole group eventually singing freely together.
2 Try this as a closing activity.

■ Relevant creative/interactive skills
Choosing a sound; listening and sharing; leading and following.

CORE ACTIVITY: VOCAL

MOUTH MUSIC

Resources: Tape recorder (if used)

■ Activity
1   Sit in a circle. It helps if the room is darkened.
2   Introduce the idea of making instrumental and rhythmic sounds with voice alone. Here are some suggestions:

    (a)   'dum', 'keh', 'tish' (bass drum, side drum and cymbal on a drum kit);

    (b)   rock guitar solo (wailing);

    (c)   'dum dum dum' (bass guitar line going up and down in pitch);

    (d)   trombone or trumpet sound (blow out cheeks and keep mouth nearly shut;

    (e)   whistling (piccolo).

3   Make up a piece with these and other sounds. You can vocalize freely or set up a backbeat with 'drum' sounds.
4   You can record the music and play it back afterwards.

NB: A number of pop songs (eg. 'Don't worry, be happy') use this technique.

■ Consideration
Break up complex sounds (like a 'drum kit' backbeat) between several players if the group finds them difficult.

■ Development
1   Try a wordless lead vocal line, or make up lyrics for it.
2   Try a 'rap' line with just rhythm sounds.
3   Try including instruments.
4   Try amplifying someone's voice through a reverberation chamber or echo unit.

■ Relevant creative/interactive skills
Depicting instrumental sounds vocally; developing the creative impulse; listening and sharing.

74

TV/FILM TASTES

Resources: TV and video, extracts from films or programmes, wallchart (if used)

■ **Activity**

1   Read 'Using video resources' (page 103) for ideas about choosing material.
2   Prepare your own material or watch what others have brought first (it may have no music or sound effects in it!).
3   Sit in a half-circle round the TV. Play a chosen film or programme extract. After watching, ask the group to share their impressions and opinions, particularly the way the music (and sound effects) fitted into the film or programme. Some suggestions:

    (a)   Did the music feel right?
    (b)   Did it fit the action?
    (c)   Did it enhance the atmosphere?
    (d)   Did it change the tone of the action or atmosphere by being there?
    (e)   Were the sound effects interesting and/or realistic?

4   You could use a wallchart to write up people's comments.
5   Play several extracts if you have time.

Tip: Reverse some of the above questions for music videos (eg. 'Did the action/atmosphere enhance the music?').

■ **Considerations**

1   See 'Listening Tastes' (page 46).
2   Visually impaired people will need to be told about the images.
3   People with a learning disability and/or a disorder of communication may find it difficult to move on from the concrete aspects of the musical/visual relationship.

■ **Development**

1   Encourage people to bring their own choice of material.
2   Move on to 'Hollywood Panel' (page 77).
3   Try 'Improvising Soundtracks 1' (page 60) and 'Improvising Soundtracks 2' (page 62).

■ Relevant creative/interactive skills

Awareness of the relationship between image and sound; listening and sharing.

HOLLYWOOD PANEL

Resources: Selection of recorded music and player, selection of videos and equipment, wallchart

■ Activity

1 Try using 'Listening Tastes' (page 46) and 'TV/Film Tastes' (page 75) before moving on to this activity.
2 Prepare video material and recorded music beforehand (see 'Using video resources' [page 103] for an example).
3 Sit in a half-circle round the TV. Watch the material together (turn off the sound) and discuss it.
4 Each time you replay the video, play one of the chosen pieces of music as a soundtrack. Ask for comments after people have watched and listened, and write these on the wallchart. Ask the group for a show of hands each time to determine the most appropriate or entertaining association of pictures and music.
5 Play the video with the sound turned up. The group will notice the re-emergence of any sound effects and dialogue. They may also find they have improved on the producer's choice of music!

Tip: You will probably need to delegate the operation of some equipment.

■ Consideration
People who feel nervous or inhibited about programme improvisation will probably find this activity more accessible.

■ Development
Try 'Improvising Soundtracks 1' (page 60), 'Improvising Soundtracks 2' (page 62), 'Directing Soundtracks' (page 63) and 'Stories' (page 64).

■ Relevant creative/interactive skills
Awareness of the relationship between image and sound; listening and sharing.

CREATIVE LISTENING FOR PERSONAL GROWTH 1

Resources: Recorded music and listening equipment

■ Activity
1   Have a choice of music ready (see 'Recorded Music' in Section 5). Use instrumental music only, as words or lyrics can engage the intellect at the expense of the listening experience. Consider a selection of around eight pieces from which you can choose. Listen to them beforehand and gauge their probable effect when heard. I suggest one piece in each of the following 'mood categories': meditative, restless, tense, angry, sad, hopeful, spiritually uplifting and relaxing (for the end of the group).
2   Sit in a circle and dim the lights. You might want to hear how people are feeling before choosing the first piece. After listening, invite the group to share their impressions and experiences.
3   Remember to warm up and wind down before and after work. Choose a slow, relaxing piece on which to end.

■ Considerations
1   Psychotherapeutic work may be unsuitable for individuals with mental health problems; if in doubt, seek the guidance of a professional practitioner.
2   People with a learning disability and/or a disorder of communication can also find it difficult to work psychotherapeutically.

■ Development
1   Consider joint work with a trained psychotherapist.
2   Consider 'Listening Tastes' (page 46) as a model for less intensive work.

■ Relevant creative/interactive skills
Translating music into experience; awareness of own needs; listening and sharing.

CREATIVE LISTENING FOR PERSONAL GROWTH 2

Resources: Recorded music and listening equipment

■ **Activity**
1   See previous activity.
2   Before listening, offer suggestions such as the following:

   (a)   the music may have a feeling or mood;
   (b)   you may be aware of your own feeling or mood when listening;
   (c)   the music may paint a picture, tell a story, or have a message that you can put into words;
   (d)   you may like, or dislike, the music;
   (e)   the music may remind you of someone;
   (f)   the music may remind you of something in your past or present, or something you anticipate in the future.

3   After listening, invite the group to share their impressions and experiences.
4   Remember to warm up and wind down before and after work. Choose a slow, relaxing piece on which to end.

■ **Considerations**
1   Psychotherapeutic work may be unsuitable for individuals with mental health problems; if in doubt, seek the guidance of a professional practitioner.
2   People with a learning disability and/or a disorder of communication can also find it difficult to work psychotherapeutically.

■ **Development**
1   Consider joint work with a trained psychotherapist.
2   Consider 'Listening Tastes' (page 46) as a model for less intensive work.

■ **Relevant creative/interactive skills**
Translating music into experience; awareness of own needs; listening and sharing.

CLOSURE: INSTRUMENTAL

COLLECTIVE HUSH

Resources: Instruments

■ Activity
1   Ask group members to choose an instrument and improvise together. You can use the suggestions in 'Free Improvisation' (page 56) before you play. Add the suggestion that, after a short time, the music will gradually become softer, and eventually fade into a thoughtful silence.
2   Hold the silence for a while after playing.

Tip: It is often positive to finish a session with silence.

■ Considerations
See 'Free Improvisation' (page 56).

■ Development
1   Try suggesting what the mood of the improvisation will be (gratitude, healing, reflection, etc).
2   Try voices, or a mixture of instruments and voices.

■ Relevant creative/interactive skills
Choosing a sound; developing the creative impulse; listening and sharing; ending.

DROP OUT

Resources: Instruments

■ Activity
1   Ask participants to choose an instrument and improvise together. You can use the suggestions in 'Free Improvisation' (page 56) before you play. After a while, ask people to drop out of the improvisation one by one (gesture is useful for this) until the sound fades into silence.
2   Hold the silence for a while after playing.

Tip: It is often positive to finish a session with silence.

■ Considerations
See 'Free Improvisation' (page 56).

■ Development
1   Try suggesting what the mood of the improvisation will be (gratitude, healing, reflection, etc).
2   Try voices, or a mixture of instruments and voices.

■ Relevant creative/interactive skills
Choosing a sound; developing the creative impulse; listening and sharing; ending.

LULLABY

Resources: Instruments

■ Activity

1 Ask people to choose instruments that will reflect the mood of a lullaby.
2 Using a metallophone (it is best tuned pentatonically: see 'Adapting instruments for maximum effectiveness' in Section 3) or similar sound source, play a simple repeated melody, setting a moderately slow to slow pulse. Invite people to join you in playing softly and gently.
3 After a while, suggest the sound will gradually become softer, then fade into a thoughtful silence.
4 Hold the silence for a while after playing.

Tip: It is often positive to finish a session with silence.

■ Consideration

Some people (especially those with a learning or physical disability) may find it difficult to sustain a rhythmic pattern or to combine it with another. Instead, try quiet 'rolled' sounds like cymbals, ocean drums or bell ropes turned gently in the hands.

■ Development

1 Real lullabies are vocal. Try a wordless solo voice or group vocalization in the spirit of the activity.
2 Ask players to 'drop out' one by one.
3 Try a freely improvised lullaby (no pulse).

■ Relevant creative/interactive skills

Choosing a sound; developing the creative impulse; listening and sharing; ending.

VOICES IN HARMONY

Resources: Keyboard (preferable) or metallophone

■ Activity

1 Darken or black out the room. You could ask people to close their eyes.
2 Start playing quietly and slowly on the black notes of the keyboard, using the sustain pedal if you have one. A setting such as 'vibes' or 'electric piano' should sound best. A metallophone with soft beaters can be used instead (it must be tuned pentatonically: see 'Adapting instruments for maximum effectiveness' in Section 3).
3 Ask group members to join in by quietly singing any note they wish (no words, just a vowel or 'la').
4 As more and more people vocalize, encourage the group to sing more freely, using two, three or more notes. Your music will give them a secure tonal framework in which to do this.
5 Let the group vocalization build and subside at its own pace; this may take several minutes. Play more softly as the end approaches, fading away to silence with the voices.
6 Allow a short silence before inviting people to open their eyes. You might leave the lights low afterwards.

Tips: Practise your style of playing beforehand. Your speaking voice needs to be clear, but relaxing. It is often positive to finish a session with silence.

■ Considerations

1 Someone who has problems with voice control may not sing in the 'key' of your music. They will not necessarily sound out of tune.
2 Some people may prefer just to listen at first.

■ Development

1 Try several tuned percussion instruments playing quiet, slow patterns.
2 Try this as a section in a larger piece.

■ Relevant creative/interactive skills

Confidence to explore and express; developing the creative impulse; listening and sharing; ending.

LISTENING AND RELAXING

Resources: Recorded music and listening equipment; floor mats (if needed)

■ Activity
1 For music ideas, see 'Recorded Music' in Section 5.
2 Sit in a circle, or lie on the floor, for this activity. It helps if the room is dimmed.
3 You can proceed in two ways:

   (a) ask people to listen and relax their minds and bodies, then play the music;
   (b) offer a guided relaxation while the music plays.

Tip: It may help to seek the advice of a skilled practitioner if you want to use guided/progressive relaxation.

■ Considerations
1 This activity may be unsuitable for people with mental health problems.
2 Some people may find the experience disturbing, or that it evokes personal feelings; they may need support.

■ Development
Try 'Listening and Visualizing' (page 87).

■ Relevant creative/interactive skills
Body awareness; awareness of own needs.

LISTENING AND VISUALIZING

Resources: Recorded music and listening equipment

■ Activity

1 See previous activity. Prepare the music beforehand and rehearse your visualization with it.
2 You might start by using 'Listening and Relaxing' (page 86) suggestions (perhaps while the music first plays).
3 Use the script below, or one based on it, to guide people through a mentally visualized experience. This should last several minutes, so speak slowly and leave lots of time in between sentences. Your voice should be clear, but relaxing.

Into the field
As you breathe deeply and relax, imagine you are in a country lane. It is a quiet, sunny day. Hear the sounds of the countryside around you; smell the grass and trees.

Walk up the lane. You see a gate into a field, and open it.

Go through the gate and walk into the field. Smell the grass and meadow flowers. Feel the grass under your feet.

You stop in the cool shade of a tree. Rest and enjoy the refreshment of the shade.

When you are rested and refreshed, walk back down the field, through the gate, back down the lane; now you are back in the room.

Remember how the experience felt. Stay with how you feel for a while.

When you are ready, open your eyes and sit (or lie) for a while.

■ Considerations

1 This activity may be unsuitable for people with mental health problems.
2 Some people may find the experience disturbing, or that it evokes personal feelings; they may need support.

■ Relevant creative/interactive skills

Body awareness; awareness of own needs.

REFLECTION AND PLANNING

Resources: Wallchart (if used)

■ Activity

1 Before you finish a group session, consider taking a little time to share and reflect on people's experiences and (if appropriate) to negotiate the activities for the next meeting. It helps to focus on what the group has achieved collectively, as well as on individually memorable moments.

2 You might invite people to share the most important experience or insight that they are taking away from the group.

3 If planning, give everyone time to contribute their ideas (including yourself). A wallchart may be useful for writing points down.

4 Thank people for taking part.

Tip: It can often be appropriate to finish a group with a short period of silence after, or even instead of, discussion. If you choose the latter, find a way to thank everyone for participating (perhaps with a quiet handshake).

IDEAS AND SKILLS TO ENHANCE YOUR WORK

Developing an instrument collection

Your group members need access to good-quality instruments covering a wide range of sounds. Avoid toy instruments as these are usually limited in scope of use, easily broken and generally age-inappropriate. I do not use them in work with children either. (Wind wands are the only exception I can think of here.) It is better to spend limited funds on just a few well-made instruments.

Some percussion instruments can be found in drum shops, but others need to be ordered from specialist retailers (see 'Equipment suppliers and dealers' in Section 5). Here is a suggested list for a small percussion collection:

▶ Cymbal on stand (16" [40cm] or 18" [45cm])
▶ Bongos (*Sonor* make good instruments)
▶ Tambourine: choose one with a head (I have found *Remo* an excellent brand)
▶ Tambour (a tambourine with no jingles)
▶ Metallophone and xylophone (these should be alto or tenor models; look at the *Sonor* catalogue)
▶ Chime bars (five will do, tuned to the black notes of the piano; try *Sonor*)
▶ Tongue drum, large (try *Knock On Wood*: see address in Section 5)
▶ Ocean drum, large (this is a frame drum with ball bearings inside; try *Knock On Wood*)
▶ Swannee whistles (there really is an *Acme* brand)
▶ Melodica (a reed instrument with piano-style keys)
▶ Bell sprays (hand-held 'jingles') and bell ropes
▶ Gong (*Paiste* have a good range)
▶ Talking drum (varies in pitch when the side cords are tightened; try *Knock On Wood*)
▶ Reed horns (these come in a set of four with interchangeable pitched reeds; contact *London Music Shop*)
▶ Wind wands (flexible tubes that 'sing' high notes when whirled round)

One very good alternative to chime bars (but more expensive) are Handchimes (*London Music Shop*). These sound rather like handbells, but in my opinion are slightly easier to use. They are gently 'thrown' forwards when played.

World percussion is a fascinating area to explore, especially African and South American instruments.

Remember beaters and sticks too.

The best kind of keyboard to buy is a small electric piano, not a home keyboard. Choose one that is loud enough to be heard without an external amplifier. Do not pay extra for 'onboard' gadgets like 'one-touch chording' unless you need them for other purposes than groupwork.

Check the portability of what you are buying, not just in case you have to transport instruments, but also because they have to be moved around in work areas.

Adapting instruments for maximum effectiveness

Tuned percussion (metallophones and xylophones)

Most of these instruments come with either diatonic (white notes of piano) or sometimes pentatonic (black note) tuned bar systems. Some (usually professional instruments) have both. You can normally remove and/or replace certain bars to alter the 'scale' in which the instrument sounds. The following are some suggestions for alternative tunings.

Diatonic

This can be a restrictive, rather than facilitative, tuning, but you might want it for (say) imitating a peal of bells. Many people find it hard to move away from 'do re mi' ideas when improvising on this scale. It is also easy to sound discordant when using it freely (try it on the piano). The notes are C D E F G A B C.

Pentatonic

Lift out all the E and B, or all the F and B, bars. This makes a useful tuning for improvisation, with no perceived discords to most ears. Many people hear this tuning as 'Chinese', but in fact it is used world-wide in many folk music traditions. The notes will be either C D F G A or C D E G A.

Whole tone

You need extra 'black notes' for this one. Tune C, D, E, F sharp, G sharp, A sharp, C and so on. Instruments often come with some of these extra bars, but you will probably need to order at least a few from your supplier. Whole-tone tuning is fascinating and 'other-worldly'; once again, discords are usually not perceived as they would be in diatonic tuning.

Harmonic minor

This is one of the 'sad' scales in Western music. It can still be restrictive, but may be more useful than straight diatonic tuning. Change all the G bars to G sharp. The notes are C D E F G sharp A B C (but the root note of this tuning would be A).

Custom tunings

My favourite is a fourths-based system: C, D, F, G, B flat, C, E flat, F, A flat and so on. Such a scale helps avoid the temptation to be 'tuneful' in a derivative way. Try your own custom tunings.

All the above are based on C as a starting-point, but can start anywhere on the chromatic (all notes) scale. There are many world tuning systems that do not even fit into Western scales; Gamelan (Indonesia) is perhaps one of the better known. Such systems can only be approximated on other instruments.

If you are confused by flats and sharps, remember:

C	sharp	=	D	flat
D	sharp	=	E	flat
F	sharp	=	G	flat
G	sharp	=	A	flat
A	sharp	=	B	flat

Do not forget to move bars along to fill in empty spaces, as this makes the instrument easier to play. It also looks less like a dentist's nightmare!

Finding notes which go well together

Start with C and G, or C and F. These two intervals (wherever they occur on the chromatic scale) are called 'perfect fifth' and 'perfect fourth', respectively; with the octave, they are the purest intervals in Western music. If heard at too low a pitch they will 'cloud' and lose their resonance.

Experiment with the pentatonic scale (above) to find notes for several instruments playing together. You can also try the whole-tone tuning, or create your own combinations of tones.

Sticks and beaters

Try building up the handles of these if they are difficult for someone to grasp. Flexible foam tubing can be useful. I once worked with a determined man who was able to use a head-pointer (a short rod attached to the front of a helmet) to play percussion.

Making instruments

It can be fun making your own instruments, but not so enjoyable trying to make music with them. They usually lack the resonance and tone of good-quality percussion. Shakers (made from containers filled with dried peas), claves (cut from brush handles) and hand drums (made by covering a balloon with papier mâché, deflating and removing the balloon, cutting the finished ball in half then using thin plastic sheeting secured with elastic for the heads) are just a few ideas.

I am enthusiastic about the possibilities of larger instruments made from recycled materials. My colleague Steve King is one of the music animateurs working in this way. I have seen him create whole 'recycled ensembles' using large plastic chemical drums placed in a circle and played with dowelling sticks; hub caps, old car springs and lengths of steel rod strung on frames (gongs and tubular bells); and a 'batphone' made from long sections of industrial plastic piping. This last instrument is played with home-made 'ping-pong bats' with rubber striking surfaces, and is tuned pentatonically by cutting the piping to certain lengths. It has a unique sound. Steve works with group composition techniques (see 'Creating a Large-Scale Piece', page 96).

'World percussion' shops have a range of literature about making ethnic instruments such as Ghanaian xylophones.

The supporter's role in improvisation

Music improvisation is a key concept, not just of music groupwork, but of music therapy. One important facilitative skill in both these areas is that of supporting and enhancing a group member's ability to create and organize sound and (in work with a therapeutic slant) to direct that ability into new areas of communicative competence and personal exploration, insight and growth. Music therapists devote much of their training to just this area of skill. Some methodologies (such as creative music therapy) favour the piano as the primary supportive instrument, while others encourage a wider range of instrumental options. In almost all, the range and application of clinical techniques is broadly similar.

Although this is in no sense a music therapy training manual, it seems useful to offer some thoughts and suggestions about supportive techniques in improvisation.

Considering the territory

I mentioned earlier (page 4) the unpremeditated nature of the act of improvising; also the way in which a person gives expression to their intent, creativity and interior psychological territory by doing so. In order to turn this from a solo activity into an interactive one, a *musical relationship* must be established. Consider the following suggestions.

Enter the territory

Listen to the way the person plays (perhaps for a few seconds at first) before joining in. The quality of their playing may be tentative or confident, interrupted or continuous, inhibited or assertive; it will have musical qualities of speed, volume, pulse, and so on. Only by listening can you first *reflect* those qualities in your own playing, then develop your reflection into *interaction*. Here your intuition guides you as much as any formal training. Interaction is the starting-point for whatever possibilities the duration of the relationship will hold. This means much more than simply mirroring what you hear: you are *responding* as a second participant and alerting your co-improviser to your presence and intent.

Explore the territory

This may (and does) happen spontaneously as you continue to be aware of each other's music. However, you can also consciously develop the style and content of the improvisation. This may happen as a partnership, or you may decide to introduce new ideas, textures or experiences. You might offer a more secure, continuous texture to frame your partner's shorter, interrupted phrases; offer new, surprising responses to playing that is rigid or perseverative; become insistently louder or suddenly softer; offer reflective pauses or silences, or match your partner's volume and energy if you feel you are being 'shut out' by uncommunicative, heavy playing. This may be consciously directive on your part, but remember that, in a partnership, both people have the freedom to offer something new. The territory belongs to both explorers.

Claim the territory together

In a truly collaborative partnership this can mean the manifestation and celebration of joint creativity, and neither of you will soon forget the experience. In a therapeutic relationship it can also mean the chance for your partner (and you!) to experience new means of self-expression, fresh areas of personal insight and growth, and new ways of communicating such insights. It can be exciting and moving to be working with someone when this happens.

It would be naïve to suggest that specialized training is not a vital component of the therapeutic supporter's ability. This does not prevent the untrained supporter exploring and appreciating the possibilities that improvisation has to offer. If the above thoughts move you to find out more about such training, then I wish you well.

Creating a large-scale piece

The individual activities and ideas in this book may be combined in many ways. It can be satisfying to create a 'larger whole' from individual pieces of creative work.

Consider 'mirror forms' when balancing the different intensity or energy of the sections. It is often aesthetically satisfying to end up as you began. In the following two examples, separate activities have been treated as episodes in a larger 'framework composition'.

Example 1

Bounce (light, fairly quiet)
Tribal Chanting (increasing energy)
Solos and Accompaniments 2 (a quieter texture and solo)
Tribal Chanting (reprise of more intense texture)
Voices in Harmony (quiet, thoughtful)

Example 2

Solos and Accompaniments 1 or *2* (quiet texture)
Building Rhythms (becoming more intense)
Mountain Tribes (in corners of room, high energy)
Building Rhythms (reprise of high energy playing)
Solos and Accompaniments (reprise of quiet texture, same soloist)

I often use episodic *Solos and Accompaniments* with three or four soloists on contrasting instruments and different supporting textures (which can include keyboard improvisation). Different textures of *Free Improvisation* can also become sections in a piece.

My colleague Steve King uses rhythms and short melodies to create group compositions. He asks members to choose five numbers, then turns them into a rhythmic sequence (for example, 1 + 5 + 4 + 2 + 7 beats), or five tones (linking the numbers to the A B C D E F G scale). They can be used in ways such as the following:

- ▶ Rhythmic phrases or repeated patterns;
- ▶ Melodies (A E D B G) or repeated patterns for tuned instruments;
- ▶ Melodic tones played in numerical sequence (A once, E five times, D four times and so on);
- ▶ Tones played together as chords in the same rhythmic sequence (once, five times, four times and so on).

He also uses pre-composed rhythm sequences for percussion, using these and other ideas to create a composition with imaginative textures and sounds (often on recycled instruments; see 'Making Instruments', above).

It is useful to plan a large-scale piece in advance, as this can inform your choice of individual ideas and activities over an extended period of time.

Arranging music from scratch

Scratch arrangements are one of the deceptively simple ideas that can enhance music groupwork. They need not (should not) be too complex, nor do they need a high level of skill to prepare. When deciding what music to arrange, ask for ideas from your group. These might be:

- ▶ favourite television or film themes
- ▶ folk songs
- ▶ pop songs (although many of these are too complex to arrange successfully)
- ▶ 'classical' tunes

The melody is your starting-point. Get to know it by listening to a recording or playing it over; sing it too.

The tune will have certain key notes, usually falling on strong beats. Note these for yourself. It helps to use music notation, but this is not vital. 'Music example 1' is an example of a tune's key notes, written first in music, then lettered, notation. These notes fall well for three reed horns; they could also be for chime bars.

Music Example 1   'Trumpet Voluntary' Key Notes

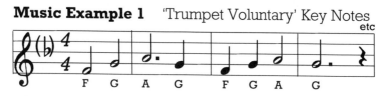

F G A G   F G A G

You might think about an accompanying line to underpin at least a part of the arrangement. In 'Music example 2' I am using two xylophone bars tuned a fifth apart.

Music Example 2   Accompanying Line

3 reed horns

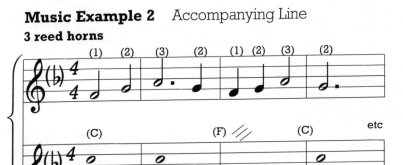

2 xylophone bars (tremolo)

Next, imagine what rhythm instruments might add: crashes on strong beats, rolls through a whole section or a regular rhythm for a while. In 'Music example 3' I have added drum and cymbal parts. If you have the skill you might try a fuller accompaniment: perhaps simple guitar or keyboard chords, or just the tune played over on a melody instrument. I usually sing the tune without accompaniment, freeing my arms to direct.

Do not put too much in (professional arrangers know that 'less means more' in terms of effect). The arrangement will be easier to play as well.

Remember this is a *blueprint*. You can change it if you want.

Music Example 3

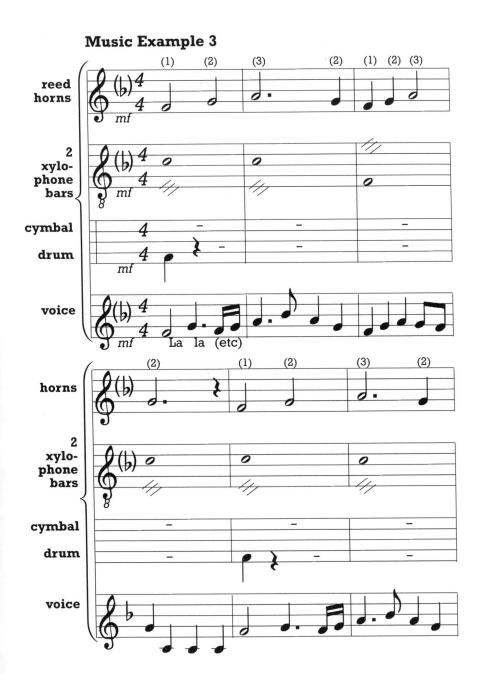

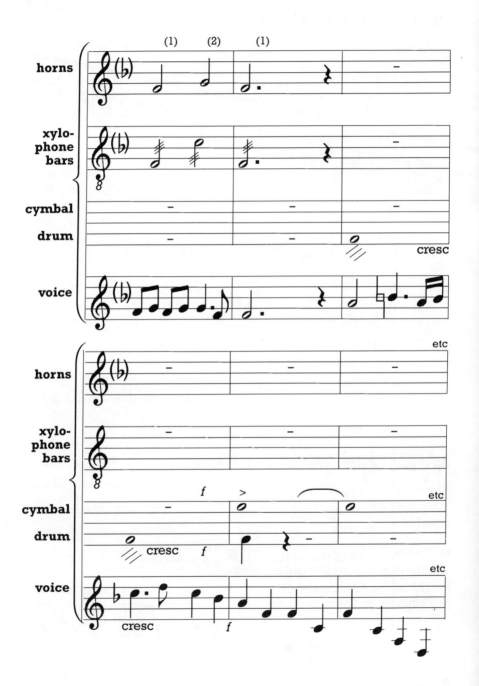

Developing skills of direction

Learn and use the eight directing gestures (see 'Basic Directing Gestures', page 52). They are almost all you will need. You will add your own style to them as you become a skilled director.

Practise bringing players in accurately 'on the beat' in a piece of music which has a pulse. To do this, try:

1 giving a warning cue by raising your arm;
2 saying "1, 2, 3, 4" (or however many beats are in the pulse); on the "4", raise your whole body slightly, lift your arm higher and cue in the strong beat with a downward gesture and motion.

After a few tries you may not need to count. It is easier to do than write about.

Practise pre-arranged cues (for example, in 'Scratch Arrangements', page 37) beforehand, so you will be confident and relaxed in the group. If you are tense and nervous, others will pick this up.

Using both arms to direct multi-instrumental work is a little like learning to drive; at first it will seem over-complicated, but as you gain skill and confidence you will be less likely to 'overload' mentally. Some people who play keyboard or guitar use head movements to direct as well.

Know your own body language: seeing yourself on video will teach you a lot about the way others read you. Finally, if you get it wrong, others will be reassured by the fact that you are only human. You can always stop, and start again.

Music and other art forms

Movement and dance

It is hard to think of a closer relationship between art forms than this one. Some ideas:

▶ Work with a dance animateur or dance/movement therapist (for therapeutic and/or artistic aims);
▶ Music and movement (for body awareness, exercise or enjoyment); it is much more effective to use live, rather than pre-recorded, music;
▶ Gentle exercise for older people (perhaps chair-based);
▶ Try incorporating movement into activities such as 'Tribal Chanting' (page 44);
▶ Directing gestures can be developed into movement/dance;

▶ *Soundbeam* is a way of controlling sound with human movement, using an ultrasonic ray which controls a synthesizer or sampler system. The range of the beam is variable to include both small and large-scale movements. This is a new musical instrument in its own right (see 'Equipment suppliers and dealers' in Section 5).

Art

Consider painting or drawing to music, which may be chosen from recordings or improvised by the group.

See 'Composing with Wallscore 1 & 2' (pages 65–6). Pictograms are artistic as well as depictive and can be developed as such.

Drama

Music can play a part in many drama groupwork activities (see **Sue Jennings**, 1986). 'Stories' (page 64) can be dramatized and plays can have 'incidental' music.

Using recording and multitrack equipment

Tape recorders

Choose good-quality equipment. Self-contained portable systems such as 'ghetto blasters' are often inferior. You need an external microphone (stereo if possible); if your machine has an internal microphone it will probably pick up motor noise too. Digital recording (like DAT) is the best of all.

For listening activities it is useful to have a remote control.

Multitrack equipment

You can record track by track on this equipment. This means you can add sounds to other sounds, then mix them together at the end. It is a very useful tool for work with 'Improvising Soundtracks 1 & 2' (pages 60–2) and other group composition activities, as you can listen to the results during the process; you can even record several versions to select from, or mix together, later. Do not get bogged down in 'retakes', though. There are a number of portable multitrack machines available, usually (at the time of writing) with the capacity to record either four or eight separate tracks. You need an amplifier and speakers when the group wants to listen to what they have recorded. Headphones are needed when listening to previous tracks while recording a fresh one; this usually means that only selected group members can hear both at the same time. Effects such as echo and reverberation can be connected to the multitrack machine.

Music recorded on some multitrack equipment at 'cassette speed' can then be played backwards on an ordinary tape recorder (see 'Quiz', page 47). Multitracking is useful when working with slides, as one of the tracks can carry the electronic 'slide change' messages for the projector.

Using video resources

When choosing material for 'TV/Film Tastes' (page 75), look for sequences where (1) music *underpins* the action; (2) music *enhances* what is happening; (3) music *transforms* what is happening. An excellent example of enhancement is Janet Leigh's drive through the the rain in *Psycho*. Two examples of transformation are the ape scene in *2001 — A Space Odyssey* and the use of Barber's 'Adagio' in *Platoon*.

When choosing material for 'Hollywood Panel' (page 77) or work with 'Improvising Soundtracks' (pages 60–2) activities, look for sequences that (1) do not rely on spoken dialogue to be understood; (2) have visual interest; (3) offer possibilities for adding sound to create atmosphere, or to enhance particular effects or events.

Early 'silents' are an interesting area to explore, as are nature films. If you are not a film buff, ask friends and family for suggestions based on the above list.

When preparing for 'Hollywood Panel', watch and get to know the sequence you will use, then decide on some key words (concepts) that describe its nature. Choose some music to match each concept. You can then find opposites or interesting/amusing alternatives to your key words, choosing other music accordingly. Pair up your pieces of music when playing them to the group. The following is an example of a list of concepts and choices:

Fight scene from *Seven Brides for Seven Brothers*
(key word) *fast* — a fast trad jazz piece,
(paired with) 'Air On A G String' (Jacques Loussier);
(key word) *dance-like* — a fast folk dance,
(paired with) 'Skaters' Waltz';
(key word) *funny* — comedy or circus music,
(paired with) Chopin's 'Funeral March';
(key word) *physical* — theme from *Rocky*,
(paired with) 'Dance of the Sugar Plum Fairy' (Tchaikovsky);

(other) — any other good ideas, such as 'Charmaine' (Mantovani version), German bierkeller music.

It is useful to have access to a wide selection of music.

SECTION 4

PARTICULAR NEEDS

Adults are not children

There are many music activity collections and educational resources for work with children. Most of these are unsuitable for adult groupwork in their published form. They include action songs, instrumental activities with song and other songs or activities which most adults would find embarrassing or irrelevant to their needs.

It is unfortunate (to say the least) that so much special needs adult music groupwork still draws on just such resources, and it is to be hoped that people become increasingly conscious of the incongruity of this in contemporary society.

As an example, consider 'picking instruments'. Children might well enjoy the idea of a 'mystery box' out of which come interesting objects to play and make sound with. Adults (or the ones I know) do not have toy boxes, and 'Open Day' (page 21) is my preferred way of exploring an instrument collection.

Another example might be an action song called 'Let's shake hands'. Here the song 'binds' and reinforces the idea of mutual greeting in a way that should appeal to children generally. It would, however, feel embarrassing or demeaning for most adults to be asked to 'de-role' and behave like children in this way. Check this for yourself when considering such an activity: how would you feel at (say) an in-service day or conference where you were asked to do this?

Here are some suggestions for your groupwork:

1   Avoid greeting, 'action' and 'activity' songs. Use voice in the ways suggested in this book: as a medium for sound exploration or (with sensitivity) in activities using the singing voice. An example of the latter would be 'Voices in Harmony' (page 84).

2   In some groupwork it will be appropriate to sing familiar songs. Many elderly people enjoy doing this together, although the tradition of community singing has been pretty well dissipated for the present generation. Most adults in our society will only sing together in certain circumstances, such as a church service or sporting event. Be sensitive to this. Do not assume that people with special needs 'love to sing'.

3   Consider the concepts of 'exploring' and 'creating' rather than 'playing' (in the childhood sense). Treat people as your equals; you are adults, engaged in jointly purposeful activity.

4   Never use an activity until you have a sense of how it will be received. Use your intuition, both when planning and when facilitating groupwork. Trust your own sense of what feels right,

and what would feel embarrassing or demeaning if you were being asked to do it yourself.

Working with elderly people

Reminiscence techniques play only a part (although an important one) in groupwork with older people. There are many issues connected with the later part of life: retirement, loss of a partner, a lifestyle increasingly dependent on others' assistance, major changes in living circumstances and the erosion of good health all spring to mind. Elderly people have always had to cope with change, but dispersed families, and a society increasingly uninterested in others' welfare, now make this even harder to do. *Personal growth* groupwork needs to take account of all this.

It can be very positive to draw a group of elderly people together by offering music for enjoyment and experience. It is important to acknowledge people's cultural norms, and activities such as 'Listening Tastes' (page 46) and 'Quiz' (page 47) should reflect this in your choice of music. As mentioned earlier, the chance to sing well-known songs (and possibly hymns) can be well received.

Many elderly people also have mental health problems, symptoms of dementia being common. When working with confused elderly people, the 'here-and-now' of individual human contact and positive relationships become central to successful groupwork. This kind of shared music activity is a worthwhile process when approached sensitively and constructively. The following are examples of two groupwork formats, the first for an enjoyment/experience group, and the second for confused elderly people.

Enjoyment/experience

Warm-up 'Listening Tastes' (15 minutes)
Core 'Open Day', 'Playing in Turn' and/or 'What's It Like?'; 'Scratch Arrangements' and/or 'Solos and Accompaniments 1' and 'Solos and Accompaniments 2' (25–30 minutes)
Closure 'Quiz' or 'Well-known Songs' or 'Voices in Harmony' (10 minutes)

For confused elderly

Warm-up 'Well-known Songs' (10 minutes)
Core 'Open Day', then individual 'Solos and Accompaniments 1' and/or 'Gamelan for Two' and/or very easy 'Scratch Arrangements'

(25–35 minutes). The supporter will usually need to play in these activities as well.
Closure 'Listening and Relaxing' (no script) (5–10 minutes)

In the second example the activities will need to be presented very flexibly, using the concepts of each core idea to engage individual members in ways which can also be shared and appreciated by others.

Working with people with a learning disability

Much has been said already about the need for a purposeful and creative approach to groupwork, rather than 'doing music' simply to fill programme time. This is never more relevant than in learning disabilities work, and groupwork for *enjoyment and experience* needs to take particular account of this (that is, not simply become a way of passing the time together). I prefer to focus on work with *creative and interactive skills* to help reinforce just such a sense of purpose. It is important to know group members' needs when planning such work, as many people with a moderate or severe learning disability also have disorders of perception or communication, or difficulty in understanding abstract concepts. Challenging behaviour may be an issue, with the chance to offer fresh opportunities for replacing negative or self-defeating behaviour with new ways of expressing oneself and interacting with others. This whole manual can be a resource for such work.

The following is an example format for work with people who have moderate to severe learning disabilities.

Warm-up 'Clap Round', then 'Open Day', 'Playing in Turn' and 'Conversations' or 'Bounce' and 'The Jungle' (20 minutes)
Core 'Solos and Accompaniments 1', then 'Solos and Accompaniments 2', or 'Directing 1', then 'Directing 2' or 'Sound Pictures 1', then 'Sound Pictures 2' (25 minutes)
Closure 'Collective Hush' (5 minutes)

Many warm-up activities can be used as core ideas too. It can be important to repeat and develop the same activities over an extended period to help people derive maximum benefit from them.

Working with people with mental health problems

Two areas are defined here: groupwork with people who are acutely (significantly and/or temporarily) ill and groupwork with those who have long-term mental health problems. The first offers opportunities for *personal growth work*, and I recommend using 'Improvising for Personal Growth 1' and 'Improvising for Personal Growth 2' and/or 'Creative Listening for Personal Growth 1' and 'Creative Listening for Personal Growth 2' as core activities, building whole groups round either or both of these ideas. These activities may not be advised for particular individuals, depending on their illness and/or circumstances. *You must seek professional guidance if at all unsure.* See the *personal growth* section in 'Planning and Running a Group: Format' (page 8), as well as the cautionary notes about these, and other, activities in Section 2.

Work in the second area might well be with *creative and interactive skills* or for *enjoyment and experience*. What I have said elsewhere about these two models also applies here (see 'Format' in 'Planning and Running a Group', page 8); the section that follows (on community work) will also be of interest.

Remember that some people may have latent symptoms when apparently in normal health: plan activities accordingly. Here is an example format:

Warm-up 'Open Day', 'What's it Like?', 'Building Rhythms' or 'Listening Tastes' (10-15 minutes)
Core 'Solos and Accompaniments 2' or 'Directing 2' and 'Directing 3' or selected instrumental warm-ups (20–25 minutes)
Closure 'Quiz' (15 minutes)

Consider carefully before using any vocal activities.

Working together: music in the community

There are now more opportunities than ever before for music groupworkers in community settings. It is worth considering some of the issues which arise here.

Integration
There is less need to offer special needs groupwork in segregated

settings, as community and arts centres open their doors to a whole range of users. Such integration can go even further. There is every reason why work for enjoyment and experience should be open to all. A common interest in music (or gentle exercise, art, drama and so on) is the best reason of all for people to get together and share such an opportunity.

New ghettos

Despite the new face of community care, perceptions and attitudes change only slowly. People with long-term mental health problems can suffer an additional burden in being labelled, 'ghettoized' or institutionalized in a way similar to the experience of many people with a learning disability. For people leaving hospital, society may have little more to offer than a transitional 'bedsit' lifestyle, a group home or perhaps a council house on a run-down estate, often close to others who have left the same institution. It is common for community services to ask arts workers to run segregated groups for such people. Consider integrating this kind of work by inviting local people to participate.

Wandering minstrels

My own peripatetic music therapy post was one of the first of its kind in Scotland and I still travel all over the Borders to work in all kinds of settings. I have been joined (here and elsewhere) by many other music workers, some of whom are clear about the aims and purpose of what they do, and others who appear to need to clarify this. It can be hard for buyers of services to judge between the merits of different offers of work. If you are a 'freelancer' (and in a sense I am too) it is important to know what you can offer and how this can be done in the best way. Consider the ideas in this manual and be clear about your strengths as well as those areas in which you need to gain expertise. Look for opportunities to share skills with service staff and seek excellence in communication with everyone in your groupwork setting; it is easy to be marginalized or misunderstood simply because you are not a full-time worker.

Good luck!

SECTION 5

RESOURCES AND CONTACTS

FURTHER READING

Ansdell G, *Music for Life: Aspects of Creative Music Therapy with Adult Clients*, Jessica Kingsley, London, 1995.

Brandon D, *Mutual Respect: Therapeutic Approaches to Working with People who have Learning Difficulties*, Good Impressions Publishing Ltd, Surbiton, Surrey, 1990.

British Journal of Music Therapy (published twice yearly).

Bruscia K, *Improvisational Models of Music Therapy*, Charles C. Thomas, Springfield, Illinois, 1987.

Bunt L, *Music Therapy: An Art Beyond Words*, Routledge, London, 1994. This is an excellent and up-to-date introduction to the subject.

Campbell J, *Creative Art in Groupwork*, Speechmark Publishing, Bicester, 1993.

Douglas T, *Basic Groupwork*, Tavistock/Routledge, London, 1988.

Green B & Gallwey T, *The Inner Game of Music*, Pan, London, 1987.

Jennings S, *Creative Drama in Groupwork*, Speechmark Publishing, Bicester, 1986.

Mathieu W, *The Listening Book: Discovering Your Own Music*, Shambhala, 1991.

Nordoff P & Robbins C, *Creative Music Therapy*, John Day, New York, 1977. This book contains useful exercises for keyboard improvisation.

Payne H, *Creative Movement and Dance in Groupwork*, Speechmark Publishing, Bicester, 1990.

Priestley M, *Music Therapy in Action*, Constable, London, 1975.

Rogers C, *On Becoming a Person*, Constable, London, 1976.

Warren B (ed), *Using the Creative Arts in Therapy: a practical introduction*, Routledge, London, 1993.

RECORDED MUSIC

As regards 'Creative Listening for Personal Growth', here are some suggestions for music in each of the eight 'mood categories' referred to on page 79. I do not recommend specific recordings in most cases, as they may not continue to be available.

Meditative

Pärt: 'Tabula Rasa'
Vaughan Williams: 'Fantasia on a Theme by Thomas Tallis'
Debussy: 'Nuages' (Nocturnes)
Tavener: 'The Protecting Veil'
Górecki: *Symphony No. 3* (the words do not detract from the atmosphere in this piece)

Restless

Holst: 'Mercury' (*The Planets*)
Stravinsky: *Rite of Spring* (opening)

Tense

Bartók: 'Music for Strings, Percussion and Celesta' (first movement)
Lutoslawski: *Cello Concerto* (opening)
Martinů: *Double Concerto for Strings and Timpani*
Stravinsky: *Petrushka* (second section)

Angry

Holst: 'Mars' (*The Planets*)
Bartók: *The Miraculous Mandarin* (central dance)
Shostakovich: *Symphony No. 4* (opening)

Sad

Mahler: 'Adagietto' (*Symphony No. 5*)
Shostakovich: *Symphony No. 5* (third movement)
Albinoni: 'Adagio'
Stravinsky: 'Berceuse' (*Firebird Suite*)
Barber: 'Adagio for Strings'

Hopeful

Horner: 'The Place Where Dreams Come True' (*Field of Dreams* film soundtrack)
Elgar: 'Nimrod' (*Enigma Variations*)

Spiritually uplifting

Delius: 'The Song of the High Hills'
Holst: 'Neptune' (*The Planets*)

Relaxing

Pachelbel: 'Canon'
Phil Thornton: 'Edge of Dreams' (New World Music)

For 'Listening and Relaxing' (page 86) and 'Listening and Visualizing' (page 87), refer to the first and the last three categories above. New age music (for example, from the New World Music catalogue) is useful.

EQUIPMENT SUPPLIERS AND DEALERS

Retailers may come and go, but I have found the following dealers invaluable:

Knock on Wood
Glasshouses Mill
Pateley Bridge
Harrogate HG3 5QH
United Kingdom
Tel 01423 712712
www.knockonwood.co.uk

Knock On Wood's catalogue of world percussion, recorded music and books is very interesting.

LMS Music Supplies
PO Box 7
Exeter
EX1 1WB
United Kingdom
Tel 01392 428108
www.LMSMusicSupplies.co.uk

LMS will supply the *Sonor* catalogue (which includes metallophones, xylophones, chime bars, bongos and so on).

For information on recording and other electronic equipment, contact:
Dawsons Music Ltd
Education Division
65 Sankey Street
Warrington WA1 1SU
United Kingdom
Tel 01925 632591
www.Dawsons.co.uk

For information on *Soundbeam*, contact:
Tim Swingler
The Soundbeam Project
Unit 3
Highbury Villas
Kingsdown
Bristol BS2 8BY
United Kingdom
Tel 0117 974 4142
www.soundbeam.co.uk

Speechmark Publishing Ltd
Telford Road
Bicester
Oxon OX26 4LQ
United Kingdom
Tel 01869 244644
Fax 01869 320040
www.speechmark.net

TRAINING AND INFORMATION

For information on music therapy training, contact:
Diana Asbridge, Administrator
Association of Professional Music Therapists
26 Hamlyn Road
Glastonbury
Somerset BA6 8HT
Tel 01458 834919
www.apmt.org.

For information about music therapy, including short courses, contact:
American Music Therapy Association, Inc.
8455 Colesville Road
Suite 1000
Silver Spring
Maryland 20910
United States of America
Tel 301 589 3300
Fax 301 589 5175
www.musictherapy.org

Denize Christophers, Administrator
British Society for Music Therapy
25 Rosslyn Avenue
East Barnet
Herts EN4 8DH
United Kingdom
Tel 0208 368 8879
www.bsmt.org

Steve King and I teach extramural courses at the University of St Andrews; contact:

Tutor in Learning Disability Training
School of Psychology
University of St Andrews
Fife KY16 9AJ
Scotland
United Kingdom
Tel 01334 476161
www.st-and.ac.uk

Sound Sense

This is an organization of community musicians from different backgrounds and in various types of work. It publishes 'Sounding Board' four times a year and organizes meetings and conferences.
Contact:
Sound Sense
7 Tavern Street
Stowmarket
Suffolk IP14 1PJ
United Kingdom
Tel 01449 673990
Fax 01449 673994
www.soundsense.org

MUSIC, VIDEO AND THE LAW

If you are using copyright material (whether published and/or recorded music or films/TV programmes and so on) in your groupwork, be aware that such use may need to be covered by up to three separate licences which should usually be purchased by the people or service who own or run the building in which you work. Here are the addresses relevant to the UK:

MCPS Media Licensing
Copyright House
29–33 Berners Street
London W1T 3AB
Tel 0207 306 4500
Fax 0207 306 4380
www.mcps.co.uk
MCPS represent composers and publishers of music

PPL
1 Upper James Street
London W1F 9DE
Tel 0207 534 1000
Fax 0207 534 1111
www.ppl.uk.com
PPL deal with sound recordings

VPL
1 Upper James Street
London W1F 9DE
Tel 0207 534 1400
Fax 0207 534 1414
www.ppl.uk.com
VPL license the use of video recordings

In the USA the NMPA's mission is to encourage understanding of copyright law so as to protect musical works against piracy and infringement. Contact them at:

Music Publishers' Association of the United States/National Music Publishers Association
PMB 246
1562 First Avenue
New York
New York 10028
United States of America
Tel/Fax 212 327 4044
www.mpa.org

Stay legal!

AFTERWORD

Please write to me if you would like to comment on anything in this manual, have any questions or just want to get in touch, at:
1 Buckholm Mill Cottages
Galashiels
Selkirkshire
TD1 2HA
United Kingdom

ALPHABETICAL LIST OF ACTIVITIES

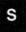

W

Creative Activities ... the Complete Series

Creative Action Methods in Groupwork
Andy Hickson
Foreword by Clive Barker
Suitable for groups of different ages and mixed genders, this excellently practical manual discusses and outlines action methods – techniques that can be used to explore difficulties or problems within the safety of a group.

Creative Art in Groupwork
Jean Campbell
Highly accessible, this manual contains 142 art activities developed specifically for use with groups of people of all ages.

Creative Drama in Groupwork
Sue Jennings
150 ideas for drama in this one practical manual make it a veritable treasure trove that will inspire everyone to run drama sessions creatively, enjoyably and effectively.

Creative Games in Groupwork
Robin Dynes
Presented in a format that immediately allows you to see what materials are needed, how much preparation is required and how each game is played, *Creative Games in Groupwork* follows the Speechmark tradition of providing practical books that are of real value to the user.

Creative Movement & Dance in Groupwork
Helen Payne
A strong link exists between movement and emotion; Helen Payne's innovative book explores that link and provides 180 practical activities with a clear rationale for the use of dance movement to enrich therapy and programmes.

Creative Music in Groupwork
Christopher Achenbach
This inspirational manual offers users effedtive ways of entering the field of music groupwork with all ages and abilities. The author sets out to share his enthusiasm with both skilled and unskilled practitioners in a manual that is wholly practical. He stresses that music groupwork is not just about therapeutic aims, but also about sharing and working creatively with others in endeavours which can be purposeful and enjoyable.

Creative Relaxation in Groupwork
Irene Tubbs
With more than 100 activities this unique text offers a goldmine of techniques and processes for relaxation.

Creative Writing in Groupwork
Robin Dynes
Here are activities designed to help participants express themselves, explore situations, compare ideas and develop both imagination and creative ability. Bursting with ideas and practical suggestions, Robin Dynes's book positively encourages creative writing as an effective activity for individuals and groups.

For further information or to obtain a free copy of the Speechmark catalogue, please contact:

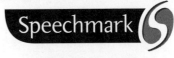

Telford Road • Bicester Oxon OX26 4LQ • UK

Tel: 01869 244644
Fax: 01869 320040
www.speechmark.net